Forensic Biomechanics

Forensic Biomechanics

Jules Kieser

Director, Sir John Walsh Research Institute, Faculty of Dentistry, University of Otago, Dunedin, New Zealand

Michael Taylor

Science Leader, Institute of Environmental Science and Research (ESR), Christchurch Science Centre, New Zealand

Debra Carr

Impact and Armour Group, Department of Engineering and Applied Science, Cranfield Defence and Security, Cranfield University, Defence Academy of the United Kingdom, Shrivenham, Wiltshire, United Kingdom

WILEY-BLACKWELL

A John Wiley & Sons, Ltd., Publication

Wiley-Blackwell is an imprint of John Wiley & Sons, formed by the merger of Wiley's global Scientific, Technical and Medical business with Blackwell Publishing.

Registered office:
John Wiley & Sons, Ltd, The Atrium, Southern Gate, Chichester, West Sussex, PO19 8SQ, UK

Editorial Offices:
9600 Garsington Road, Oxford, OX4 2DQ, UK
The Atrium, Southern Gate, Chichester, West Sussex, PO19 8SQ, UK
111 River Street, Hoboken, NJ 07030-5774, USA.

For details of our global editorial offices, for customer services and for information about how to apply for permission to reuse the copyright material in this book please see our website at www.wiley.com/wiley-blackwell The right of the author to be identified as the author of this work has been asserted in accordance with the UK Copyright, Designs and Patents Act 1988.

Library of Congress Cataloging-in-Publication Data

Kieser, Jules.
  Forensic biomechanics / Jules Kieser, Michael Taylor, Debra D. Carr.
     p. ; cm.
  Includes bibliographical references and index.
  ISBN 978-1-119-99011-6 (hardback)
  I. Taylor, Michael, 1953 Sept. 18-   II. Carr, Debra D.   III. Title.
  [DNLM: 1.   Biomechanics. 2.   Forensic Sciences–methods. 3.   Wounds and Injuries–pathology. W 750]
  617.1–dc23

                                                                                              2012027882

A catalogue record for this book is available from the British Library. Wiley also publishes its books in a variety of electronic formats. Some content that appears in print may not be available in electronic books.

Set in 10.5/13pt Times-Roman by Thomson Digital, Noida, India
First Impression 2013

This book is dedicated to Glynny Kieser, who first suggested it, oversaw every stage of its production and kept our team together.

Contents

Series Foreword

The world of forensic science is changing at a very fast pace in terms of the provision of forensic science services, the development of technologies and knowledge and the interpretation of analytical and other data as it is applied within forensic practice. Practicing forensic scientists are constantly striving to deliver the very best for the judicial process and as such need a reliable and robust knowledge base within their diverse disciplines. It is hoped that this book series will provide a resource by which such knowledge can be underpinned for both students and practitioners of forensic science alike.

It is the objective of this book series to provide a valuable resource for forensic science practitioners, educators and others in that regard. The books developed and published within this series come from some of the leading researchers and practitioners in their fields and will provide essential and relevant information to the reader.

Professor Niamh Nic Daéid
Series editor

Acknowledgements

One of the most rewarding things about writing this book has been the privilege of reading the writings of so many of our colleagues, past and present. This book rests heavily on the shoulders of other books and hundreds upon hundreds of scientific articles that have been penned on the subject; many of which are referenced in the text. It also rests upon the hard work of our under- and post-graduate students over the years. This book would have been impossible without the inspiration of these young people, who continued to challenge and teach us as we wrote. We stand in their debt.

This book is also heavily indebted to forensic scientists of all persuasions. We know a few of them professionally and we hope that their views have not been misrepresented. We owe much to Michael Swain for his painstaking editing of aspects of this book, and to his collaboration and advice to us over many years. Special thanks are also due to those who had the stamina and good humour to read through and comment on parts of the manuscript: Darryl Tong and Neil Waddell.

There are many forensic pathologists, forensic scientists, odontologists and members of diverse law enforcement agencies who independently worked with us or talked to us confidentially; including some who gave most generously of their time and hospitality. These include Michael Tsokos, Jane Taylor, Antony Hill, Stephen Knott, Richard Bassed, Hugh Trengrove, Ross Meldrum, Norman Firth, Warwick Duncan, Maryna Steyn, David Kieser, Raj Das and Gemma Dickson. We thank them all. For images and illustrations we thank Liz Girvan (scanning electron micrographs), Andrew McNaughton (micro-computed tomography) and Matt Blair (drawings).

All errors and wrong interpretations are, of course, our responsibility alone. It has been our decision not to write in legalese or scientific jargon. May the pedantic academics forgive us.

How does one thank the most important people of all? Fiona Seymour, Rachael Ballard and Izzy Canning, all at John Wiley & Sons, Ltd. A special word of thanks to Clare Lendrem, our copy-editor extraordinaire, whose professionalism goes unmatched. Glynny Kieser collated, edited and prepared the manuscript.

1
Introduction

Jules Kieser

In solving a problem of this sort, the grand thing is to be able to reason backward. That is a very useful accomplishment, and a very easy one, but people do not practise it much.

Sir Arthur Conan Doyle: *A Study in Scarlet* (2010, p. 83)

Biomechanics has its own terminology that is based upon that of mechanical engineering. The translators of the code of biomechanics are the engineers who have developed their own jargon. It is our intent to reveal some of the fundamentals of biomechanical testing and many specific testing techniques. In so doing, we hope to disperse the mystique shrouding biomechanics.

Turner and Burr (1993, p. 595)

Biomechanics is a new, exciting and powerful discipline that is shaping a broad range of subjects such as medicine, sports science, botany, zoology, ergonomics, accident reconstruction, occupational health, palaeobiology, dentistry and, most recently, forensics. Many of these areas have developed sophisticated biomechanical techniques with their own algorithms, notation and specialised methods. This combination of breadth and depth makes it impossible for any one individual to master all of the biomechanical approaches that have been developed. The aim of this book is thus twofold; it introduces general concepts that apply to the field as a whole, and it applies these to the broad discipline of forensic biology.

Whereas it is difficult to identify a father of biomechanics, one could argue that biomechanics is as old as mechanics itself. The Italian renaissance scientist, Leonardo da Vinci (1452–1519) studied the biomechanics of the flight of birds and, by extension, hypothesised how humans could fly. Galileo Galilei (1564–1642) investigated the strength of bones and suggested that they were hollow, because this gave them a maximum strength for minimum weight. Rene Descartes (1596–1650) proposed a philosophical view that saw all material systems, including the human body, as machines ruled by simple mechanical laws; an idea that did much to promote and sustain the biomechanical studies of Giovani Borelli (1608–1679) and others (for review, see Humphrey, 2003).

The term *Biomechanics* itself has only recently been defined by the South African scientist Herbert Hatze (1937–2002) as 'the study of the structure and function of biological systems by means of the methods of mechanics' (Hatze, 1974, p. 189). He

Forensic Biomechanics, First Edition. Jules Kieser, Michael Taylor and Debra Carr.
© 2013 John Wiley & Sons, Ltd. Published 2013 by John Wiley & Sons, Ltd.

was at pains to stress that, because biological systems cannot have mechanical aspects, one cannot apply pure mechanics to such systems. By way of example, consider the trajectory, velocity, spin, angle of impact etc. of a bullet striking a living target. Before impact, the simple laws of mechanics govern all aspects of the projectile's travel. The situation changes immediately upon impact: we now have to draw on vastly more complex biomechanical aspects of the tissues involved to interpret the resultant pattern of wounding, path of travel, bloodspatter and so on. In this book, we accept *forensic biomechanics as the study of forensic biological phenomena by means of the methods of mechanics, in terms of the structure and function of relevant biological systems.*

Modern biomechanics had its roots in the 1970s, when digital computers became more generally available and when the *International Society of Biomechanics* was founded. A key pioneering publication was that of *Biomechanics: Mechanical Properties of Living Tissues* by Y. C. Fung (1993), who characterised the field as mechanics applied to biology. With the application of rigorous engineering analyses to the study of biological tissues in the seventies and eighties came the realisation that conventional mechanical methods were generally inadequate to model biological tissues. Bone, for instance, behaved in a linearly elastic fashion, and yet it was anisotropic, with mechanical properties dictated by its micro- and macroarchitecture. Skin and other soft tissues exhibited anisotropic viscoelasticity, and blood was found to behave in a non-Newtonian fashion. These behaviour patterns required a new set of theoretical frameworks, motivated by observations in living tissues, which in turn were subjected to more observation, using increasingly sophisticated methods such as scanning electron microscopy, nano-indentation and micro-CT (micro-computed tomography) scanning (Athesian and Friedman, 2009). Additionally, biomechanics was being applied to multiscale systems consisting of bodies, organs, cells and subcellular structures. To facilitate this, a multidisciplinary integrative approach, ranging from biophysics of molecules to bulk constitutive modelling, had to be developed. While forensic biology research is clearly evident at the tissue and organ level, it can and does involve several levels of hierarchy and, hence, forensic biomechanics is application focused and relies on basic biomechanical knowledge at all levels from nano- to whole body structures. Improved understanding of the role of biomechanics in the broad field of forensics will lead to new investigative approaches that will strengthen the evidentiary usefulness of forensic science in general.

We offer no apology for adding another text to the forensic science library. Our intention is simply to make the biomechanical principles of forensic biology more relevant and understandable. While making a humble contribution to the subject, this book is designed to meet the pressing need for an overall description of biomechanical principles that does not require background knowledge of mathematics. Many of us find formulae, particularly the longer ones that employ Greek symbols, daunting and incomprehensible. Most people understand basic laws of motion and relationships between factors such as stress and strain, but when faced with their shorthand mathematical expressions we experience an attention deficit problem. Unfamiliarity with algebra and calculus lie at the root of this. Here, we overcome this issue by using clarity of writing and simple examples. In doing so, we obviously risk irritating those more familiar with higher mathematical skills such as linear algebra, calculus and Fourier transforms, and we apologetically refer them to those more involved texts that might suit their needs better. Hence, the basic premise of this book is that most forensic biological principles can be understood and used without the traditional barriers of higher mathematics and theory. We wish to emphasise that this book is intended to serve a distinctly humble purpose; it introduces biomechanical principles that are useful in understanding or interpreting some forensic evidence such as trauma, bloodstain patterns and damage to natural fibres and fabrics.

The structure of the book as a whole will be evident from a glance at the table of contents. Chapter 1 introduces the subject of biomechanics and places it in the context of forensic biology. The fundamental guiding principles that are key to understanding forensic biomechanics are presented in a clear, step-by-step fashion in Chapter 2. Whether you have a mathematical background or not, this will provide you with a new and interesting perspective on forensic investigation. While the biomechanics of bone and bony trauma is the subject of Chapter 3, skin and soft tissue trauma are covered in Chapter 4. The intention of both these chapters is to provide a basic overview of the structures and processes involved, not to spend an inordinate amount of time on mathematical details. Chapter 5 describes the biomechanics of bloodspatter from the viewpoint of the forensic investigator, showing the physical principles underlying bloodstain pattern formation. Chapter 6 describes the architecture of natural fibres, yarns and fabrics and discusses how these are affected by blunt, sharp and ballistic impacts.

A modest mathematical/physics background is required to understand the material presented here. The reader is expected to have a basic understanding of physics and to be familiar with biological structures such as cells and tissues. Readers do not need sophisticated mathematics, nor do they need to know the details of kinetics, ballistics or viscoelastic, or non-Newtonian behaviour.

The book is now in the hands of its most important critic: you. Your criticisms, comments and suggestions are very important to the continued evolution of this work. All it takes is a three-minute email to jules.kieser@otago.ac.nz. Thank you so much, we hope you enjoy this book.

References

Athesian GA, Friedman MH. 2009. Integrative biomechanics: a paradigm for clinical applications of fundamental mechanics. *Journal of Biomechanics* **42**:1444–51.

Doyle AC. 2010. *Sherlock Holmes*. Penguin Books, New Delhi.

Fung YC. 1993. *Biomechanics: Mechanical Properties of Living Tissues*. Springer, Berlin.

Hatze H. 1974. The meaning of the term 'biomechanics'. *Journal of Biomechanics* **7**:189–90.

Humphrey JD. 2003. Continuum biomechanics of soft biological tissues. *Proceedings of the Royal Society London A* **459**:3–46.

Turner CH, Burr DB. 1993. Basic biomechanical measurements of bone: a tutorial. *Bone* **14**:595–608.

2
Basic principles of biomechanics

Jules Kieser

2.1   Forces and motion

Newton's laws

It is perhaps fitting to start this section with Sir Isaac Newton's (1642–1727) three laws. Hopefully, this will introduce most of the essential basics of kinetics, before we wade towards the deeper end of this chapter. There are different approaches one might take to these cardinal laws; here we will focus on their applications to biomechanics, while keeping mathematics to a minimum. Essentially, there are two assumptions upon which Newton's theory rests; the first is the concept of equilibrium and the second is the conservation of energy. Think of equilibrium as an ideal situation in which there are a number of forces acting on a point, but because the sum of the forces is zero, no change in position or velocity occurs. Take Figure 2.1 for instance. Here point **a** is stable, or in static equilibrium, because the sum of the four forces acting on it is zero. Newton's second principle is simply this: energy can neither be created nor destroyed; it can only be converted from one form to another.

Newton's first law (the law of inertia) asserts that every object at rest or in a state of uniform motion will remain in that state, unless an external force is applied to it. A body's resistance to change in motion is its inertia. What this means is that a static body has an inertia proportional to its mass: the larger the mass, the greater the force (push or pull) required to get it moving. Linear inertia is similar: it is a body's resistance to a change in its motion. There is also a rotational counterpart to the first law. The mass moment of inertia is proportional to the distribution of the mass around the axis of rotation, as well as the total mass of the object. In other words, there is increased resistance to a change in rotation if the mass is further from the axis of rotation. Hence, a roundhouse punch has a harder impact than a jab. The opposite is also true – think of an ice-skater spinning with spread arms. As she brings them together, her angular velocity increases.

Newton's second law (the law of acceleration) states that a force (F) applied to a body of mass m will cause an acceleration (a) of that body, of a magnitude proportional to the force, in the direction of that force, and inversely proportional to the body's mass, giving possibly the most widely known of all mathematical expressions:

$$F = ma$$

Forensic Biomechanics, First Edition. Jules Kieser, Michael Taylor and Debra Carr.
© 2013 John Wiley & Sons, Ltd. Published 2013 by John Wiley & Sons, Ltd.

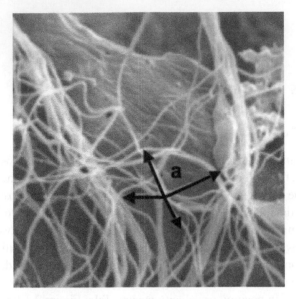

Figure 2.1   Static equilibrium on point **a** when the sum of the forces acting on it is zero.

Perhaps more importantly, it also defines the critical biomechanical concept of momentum. Momentum is a vector (it has magnitude and direction; a static body has no momentum) given as mass times velocity. When a moving object such as a fist collides with a jaw, momentum changes over a very short period of time, with a high probability of injury. However, if the fist is in a boxing glove and the punch remains the same, momentum is lost over a period of time (while the blow is cushioned by the foam in the glove), markedly lowering the probability of injury.

Newton's third law (the law of reaction) simply states that for every action there is an equal and opposite reaction. This is another critically important concept in biomechanics. When two objects interact (e.g. a fist and a jaw), action and reaction forces of equal magnitude act on the objects in opposite directions. While the action and reaction forces are equal, their effects can be spectacularly different simply because of their material differences. Think, for instance, of a steel knuckleduster impacting a jaw. A force is generated from the knuckleduster to the jawbone, and the jaw exerts an equal and opposite force on the knuckleduster. However, the effects of the interaction are disastrous for the jaw, as the material properties of steel are so vastly different from those of bone.

One point raised by Newton's laws deserves clarification: that of movement. It is important to remember that there are two forms of motion: linear and angular. *Linear motion* (translation) is movement either in a straight line (rectilinear motion) or in a curved line (curvilinear motion). *Angular motion* involves rotation about an axis. Importantly, many movements that are significant to forensics involve both; the motion of a swinging punch involves linear motion of the fist, but angular motion of the shoulder and trunk. Similarly, a bullet follows a slightly curvilinear path, but because of the rifling in the barrel, it also rotates about its own long axis.

Energy

We all know intuitively what energy is; some people have a lot of it, some don't. Without it, nothing can move and nothing gets done. Countries spend millions acquiring it, and even go to war for it. Yet it was only in the mid-19th century that the concept was defined and links between its different sub-types established. It was the British brewer, James Prescott Joule (1818–1889) who first formulated our ideas about energy, heat and work done.

At its simplest level, forensic biomechanics views energy from the point of forces and distances. The units of energy thus become similar to the technical definition of energy often used by physicists:

$$\text{Work} = \text{Force} \times \text{Distance}$$

Force is commonly described using a unit of measurement known as a newton, which is equal to the force needed to accelerate a mass of one kilogram, one metre in one second (in a vacuum with no friction). The work or energy required to move an object with the force of one newton over a distance of one metre is referred to as a joule. Hence, energy is the ability to do work, while work is the transfer of energy. Joule also established that heat was a form of energy and that the various forms of energy were basically the same and could be changed from one to another; a discovery that formed the basis of the law of conservation of energy, the first law of thermodynamics.

Momentum

The concept of momentum comes to us from the French philosopher Rene Descartes (1596–1650). Descartes stated that objects in motion had momentum, and that the amount of motion for a moving body was the product of the mass (m) of the body and its speed (s):

$$p = ms$$

Clearly, momentum is a vector: it has a size and a direction. It fell to the Dutch mathematician Christiaan Huygens (1629–1695) to figure out the effect of the momentum of two moving objects, acting in opposite directions, and to change Descartes' formula to:

$$p = mv$$

where v is the velocity.

Recall that Newton's second law states that:

$$F = ma$$

Because acceleration is the rate of change of velocity, for an object with a constant mass the formula becomes:

$$F = \text{Rate of change of momentum}$$

Consider a collision between two objects, A and B. From Newton's third law, the force that A experiences from B is of equal magnitude, but opposite in direction to the force B experiences from A. Since force is the rate of change of momentum, it follows that during the impact process the rate of change of momentum of A is exactly opposite to the rate of change of momentum of B. Hence, for every bit of momentum A gains, B gains its negative. In other words, B loses momentum at the same rate that A gains it; thus their total momentum remains the same. This holds for the entire process, from beginning to end.

The significance of this is that we already know that, because Newton's laws are obeyed throughout, and that momentum will be conserved, then, for example if A and B stick together after the impact, and no bits fly off, one can calculate their final velocity just from momentum conservation, without knowing details of the collision.

2.2 Stress and strain

One does not have to be an engineer to make some sense of the biomechanical background to forensics (we all drive vehicles without an understanding of the physics behind internal combustion), but some familiarity with physics is essential. Biomechanics of skin and bones is often more concerned with macrostructural responses than microstructural ones. The two are different, yet united in their being living tissues. Hence, collagen and its matrix may not be representative of an entire bone, such as the femur. On the other hand, one could focus on the material properties of a single collagen fibril and not even consider its ground substance. Similarly, biomechanical properties or behaviours can be measured in two- or three-dimensional space. In this section, we will discuss basic biomechanical behaviour phenomenologically, without discussing the detailed mathematics behind different concepts.

The first of these concepts that we need to look at is the one of *displacement*. Displacement is simply the shifting of a structure in response to an external force. Think of a trampoline. When you jump on a trampoline, its elastic base is displaced downwards in response to the magnitude of the force you exert onto it. Obviously, the displacement is dependent on the elasticity (stretchiness) of the fabric, and on the springs that radiate from it onto the frame. Even the frame will have at least some elasticity or give to it. If you were now to paint a grid over the trampoline, jump on it and take a high-speed photo of the maximum stretch, you could measure the displacement within each square relative to its neighbours. This change in relative position relative to an external force is the *field of displacement*. This, for example, we shall see is useful when considering blowback in ballistic injuries.

The next concept is that of *stress*. Stress is simply a measure of force acting over an area, symbolised by sigma ($\sigma = F/a$) and is measured in pascals (Pa), defined as $1\,\text{Pa} = 1\,\text{N/m}^2$. There are three broad types of stress (Fig. 2.2); normal stresses are either *compressive* or *tensile*, or, when the forces act parallel or tangential to one another, *shear* stress. In tissue mechanics, stress is mostly measured in megapascals ($1\,\text{MPa} = 1\,\text{N/mm}^2$). Typically tensile strength and compressive strength are terms applied to a material's resistance to stretching or crushing. Materials often differ in their abilities to withstand tensile or compressive loads.

Strain is a measure of shape change or deformation and is always measured in relative terms. Strain, given as epsilon ε, is measured as the change in dimension resultant from an external force, divided by the resting dimension; in other words $\varepsilon = \Delta l/l$. Strain is dimensionless, and is often reported as a percentage, and can be either normal – in other words, compressive or tensile – or it can be shear. In biological tissues strains can be very small, and are then reported as microstrain – $\mu\varepsilon$ – with $1000\,\mu\varepsilon$ being 0.1% (0.001).

Stresses and strains can of course be considered in three dimensions, which makes things rather difficult. A cube, for instance, consists of six squares (three pairs or mirror images); hence $3 + 3 + 3 + 9$ strains.

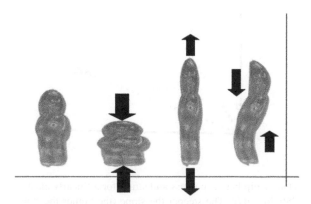

Figure 2.2 A jelly baby subjected to compressive, tensile and shear stress.

The relationship between stress and strain: there is a unique relationship between stress (force) and strain (deformation), referred to as the constitutive law of the material being stressed. In some isotropic, non-biological materials such as a steel spring, the stress/strain relationship is a straight line. This linear relationship is described by Hooke's law, which states simply that the strain experienced by a material is directly proportional to the applied stress. This ratio is known as *Young's modulus*, or the modulus of elasticity E (named after Thomas Young, the English polymath, 1773–1829).

Hence, $E = \text{Stress}/\text{Strain} = \sigma/\varepsilon$. Materials that behave in this way are referred to as linearly elastic. Ductile materials such as soft gold or rubber have low Young's moduli (Fig. 2.3), and stiff materials such as glass have high Young's moduli.

Elasticity implies non-permanent deformation during loading. In other words, when the load is removed, the materials recover their original shape. Some materials behave in this fashion only until they are loaded beyond a given point. At higher loads, they do not recover, but deform permanently. This point is called the *elastic limit*, and after it is reached deformation is said to be *plastic* (permanent). In contrast to elastic deformation, plastic deformation is irreversible (Fig. 2.4). In reality, an elastic deformation is superimposed on any plastic deformation so that the elastic part of the deformation will revert, but the plastic part remains. For this reason, one important problem in investigating the deformation of materials is to distinguish between elastic and plastic parts of the strain.

Similar to elastic deformations, plastic deformations can be time dependent or time independent. The term plasticity always implies time-independent deformation.

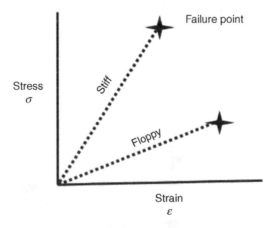

Figure 2.3 The relationship between stress and strain for a linearly elastic material, Young's modulus $E = \text{Stress}/\text{Strain} = \sigma/\varepsilon$. The steeper the slope (the higher the Young's modulus), the stiffer the material. The smaller the Young's modulus, the less stiff or the more floppy it is.

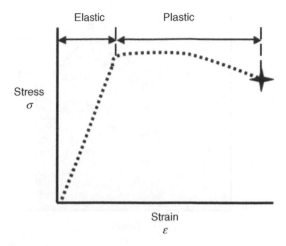

Figure 2.4 Stress/Strain curve showing a linear elastic response, followed by plastic deformation and eventual failure.

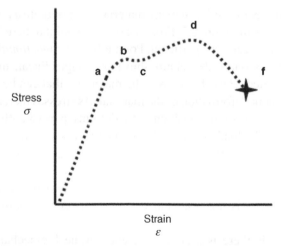

Figure 2.5 Schematic representation of the stress/strain relationship for biological tissues. Point **a** represents the *proportional limit* beyond which the relationship is no longer linear, but elastic. Point **b** is the *elastic limit*, which is the maximum stress that can be applied without resulting in permanent deformation of the material. As stresses increase, the material deforms permanently: *plastic deformation*. Point **c** is the *yield point* at which elongation (yielding) can occur with relatively little increased stress. At point **d**, the highest point on the stress/strain curve is reached, where the material reaches its *ultimate strength* before failing. Failure in most tissues is not instantaneous, and occurs at a variable point, **f**.

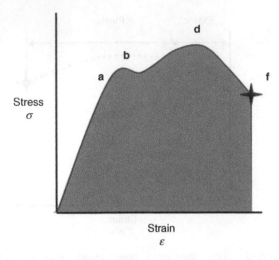

Figure 2.6 Schematic representation of the stress/strain relationship for biological tissues, showing the area under the curve, which when divided by the volume of the material is a measure of the strain energy density.

Time-dependent plastic deformation is *viscoplasticity or creep* (Chailleux and Davies, 2003).

The stress/strain relationships in many materials are not quite as simple. Consider the stress/strain curve in Figure 2.5. From the origin to point **a** there is a straight line; stress and strain are linearly proportional. Point **a** is the *proportional limit*. As stress increases beyond this point, the relationship is no longer linear, until point **b**, the *elastic limit*, is reached. Here the stress is the maximum that can be applied without resulting in permanent deformation of the material. As stresses increase, the material ceases to behave in an elastic fashion, and deforms permanently, called *plastic deformation*. When the load is removed, the material does shorten again, but not to its original size. Point **c** is the *yield point* at which elongation (yielding) can occur with relatively little increased stress. At point **d**, the highest point on the stress/strain curve, the material reaches its *ultimate strength*, beyond which it starts failing. Failure in most tissues is not instantaneous, and it occurs at point **f**, the point of rupture.

In many materials there is a large difference in the biomechanical behaviour, depending on the directionality of the applied force. When these properties vary with different loading orientations, the material is said to be *anisotropic*. Alternatively, when the material properties are the same in all directions, the material is *isotropic*. Most biological materials behave in an anisotropic fashion.

A final important note is that the area under the stress/strain curve is a measure of the strain energy stored within the tissue prior to failure, or the *strain energy density* (Fig. 2.6).

Poisson's ratio

When you squeeze a jelly baby, it gets fatter (Fig. 2.2). One person to make a major contribution to our understanding of the behaviour of materials under load was the French mathematician Simeon Denis Poisson (1798–1840). He described the phenomenon that when a material is compressed in one direction, it tends to expand in the other two directions perpendicular to the direction of compression. This is called the Poisson effect. Poisson's ratio v (nu), simply a measure of this effect, is the ratio of the percentage (or fraction) of expansion divided by the percentage (or fraction) of compression. Hence, $v = -(\varepsilon_t/\varepsilon_a)$, where ε_t is the tangential strain and ε_a is the axial strain. The reason why this is so, is that most materials resist a change in volume more than they resist a change in shape. The opposite is also true; when a material is stretched, its dimensions contract at right angles to the pulling force and Poisson's ratio becomes the ratio of transverse contraction strain (deformation) to longitudinal extension strain (deformation) in the direction of the stretching force. Tensile deformation is considered positive, and compressive deformation is considered negative. The Poisson's ratio of an isotropic, linear elastic material cannot be less than -1.0 nor greater than $\frac{1}{2}$ (0.5) due to the requirement that Young's modulus, the shear modulus and bulk modulus have positive values (most materials have Poisson's ratios between 0.0 and 0.5). Physically the reason is that, for a material to be stable, its stiffness must be positive; the bulk and shear stiffness are interrelated by formulae that incorporate Poisson's ratio (Sokolnikoff, 1983). A practical example of the application of a particular value of Poisson's ratio is the cork of a wine bottle, which has to be easily inserted and removed, but must also withstand pressure from within the bottle. In contrast, rubber has a Poisson's ratio of 0.5 and will expand when pushed into the neck of the bottle and would jam.

2.3   Basics of biomechanical behaviour

Biomechanical behaviour of tissues such as bone, skin or teeth subjected to different forces and moments is not only affected by the mechanical properties discussed above, but also by factors such as the geometry of the impacted structure, the mode of force application, and its direction, rate and frequency.

Biomechanics is essentially a practical theory. It gives physical meaning to the biological and mechanical behaviour of the tissues that comprise a living being, and how these interact in response to normal or abnormal forces brought to bear on them. It is one thing to know something of how simple unidirectional loading of a biological material works, but what about the more realistic situation of bi- or multidirectional loading? Let us firstly consider loading in two directions.

Case 2.1   Limitations of forensic biomechanics

Forensic biomechanical evidence is clearly intended for court presentation. However, while forensic biomechanics has been most useful in explaining how observed injuries occurred, it may be less valuable in the evaluation of competing hypothetical interpretations of an observed traumatic event (Freeman and Kohles, 2011). This case illustrates the point. Clearly, the person here had died as a result of hanging. Determining the cause is a biomechanical exercise in that it can be attributed to a 'hangman's fracture' of the axis of second cervical vertebra, cerebral ischaemia resultant from compression of the vertebral or carotid arteries, or to decapitation. Whether this was dependent upon the type of knot, the thickness of the rope or the length of drop on the one hand, or to body mass or body position on the other, is highly dependent on the complexity of the anatomy and physiology of the neck.

The result is that forensic biomechanical analysis has tended to use mathematical modelling on experimentally derived data to show that those forces involved in a particular trauma event, such as hanging, were sufficient to cause death. On the other hand, interpretation of biomechanical plausibility of the exact cause of death has not been as successful.

Reference

Freeman MD, Kohles SS. 2010. Applications and limitations of forensic biomechanics: a Bayesian approach. *Journal of Forensic and Legal Medicine* *17*:67–77.

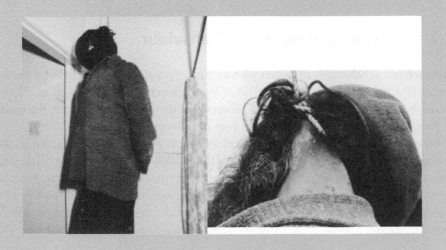

Two-directional loading: Figure 2.7 shows a rectangular shape being loaded in two directions (F_x and F_y), resulting in stresses along the x-axis of $\sigma_x = F_x/a_x$, and the y-axis of $\sigma_y = F_y/a_y$. Of course, the stresses will result in elongation and thinning according to Poisson's theorem. Remembering that Poisson's ratio is $v = -(\varepsilon_t/\varepsilon_a)$, and that Hooke's law states that stress $\sigma = E \cdot \varepsilon$, we now have that directional strains attributable to σ_x are

$$x\text{-axis}: \varepsilon_{x\sigma_x} = \sigma_x/E \text{ and } y\text{-axis}: \varepsilon_{y\sigma_x} = -v \cdot (\sigma_x/E)$$

Similarly, strains attributable to σ_y are

$$y\text{-axis}: \varepsilon_{y\sigma_y} = \sigma_y/E \text{ and } x\text{-axis}: \varepsilon_{x\sigma_y} = -v \cdot (\sigma_y/E)$$

Combined, the net strains along the two axes now become:

$$\varepsilon_x = \varepsilon_{x\sigma_x} + \varepsilon_{x\sigma_y} = (\sigma_x/E) - v \cdot (\sigma_y/E)$$

and

$$\varepsilon_y = \varepsilon_{y\sigma_y} + \varepsilon_{y\sigma_x} = (\sigma_y/E) - v \cdot (\sigma_x/E)$$

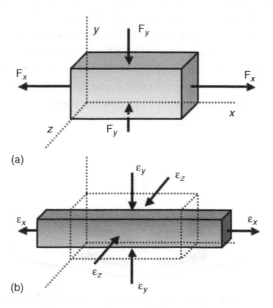

(a)

(b)

Figure 2.7 (a) A rectangular shape being loaded in two directions (F_x and F_y), resulting in stresses along the x-axis of $\sigma_x = F_x/a_x$, and the y-axis of $\sigma_y = F_y/a_y$. (b) Resultant elongation is shown in the shaded figure. Combined net strains along the two axes are $\varepsilon_x = \varepsilon_{x\sigma_x} + \varepsilon_{x\sigma_y} = (\sigma_x/E) - v \cdot (\sigma_y/E)$ and $\varepsilon_y = \varepsilon_{y\sigma_y} + \varepsilon_{y\sigma_x} = (\sigma_y/E) - v \cdot (\sigma_x/E)$ respectively.

Three-directional loading results from an additional load in the z-axis, with the mathematical expressions becoming too complicated for this introductory text.

Material behaviour during bending

When an elongated structure, such as a long bone, is loaded perpendicular to its long axis, it bends (Fig. 2.8). The outer, convex surface will experience tensile stress, while the inner, concave surface experiences compressive stress. Although both Galileo and Bernoulli have been credited with being the 'fathers' of beam theory, it was not until fairly recently that it was realised that Leonardo da Vinci's work (published in 1493) correctly identified stress and strain distributions across a beam during bending. Importantly, these scientists recognised that the tensile and compressive stresses are at a maximum on the outer surfaces of the structure being bent, and that the material at its centre (the neutral axis) experiences no stress at all.

How a structure such as a beam (Fig. 2.8) resists bending is largely dependent on its elastic modulus, together with the moment arm and the moment of area (second moment of area). The moment of area depends on the cross-sectional area of the beam and how it is dispersed around a reference axis. The larger the moment of area, the less the beam will bend (see Section 3.4). This leaves the moment arm. Also known as the lever arm, it simply refers to the fact that the magnitude of a force about a point is equal to the magnitude of that force, multiplied by the length of the shortest distance between the line of action of the force and the point of application. It follows that the dimension of the moment is the dimension of the force times the dimension of the moment arm length (e.g. newton-metre, N·m).

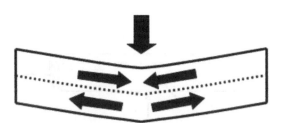

Figure 2.8 The behaviour of an elongated structure loaded perpendicular to its long axis. As it bends, the outer, convex surface experiences tensile stress and the inner, concave surface experiences compressive stress. While tensile and compressive stresses are at a maximum on the outer surfaces of the structure, the material at its centre (the neutral axis – dotted line) experiences no stress.

2.4 Biomaterials and viscoelasticity

In the late 19th century, scientists such as James Clerk Maxwell (1831–1879) and Lord Kelvin (1824–1907) started looking at some naturally occurring materials, for instance tar or dough, that flow over time. When such materials were subjected to a constant load, they did not show a constant deformation (as Hooke's law would predict). Instead, these substances could clearly be seen to flow while loaded; a phenomenon referred to as *creep*. As soon as the load was removed, a noticeable recovery occurred until the original dimensions were eventually regained. This phenomenon of creep under load was clearly neither a plastic nor an elastic response, but rather a 'delayed elasticity' or an 'elastic after-effect' (for discussion see Markovitz, 1977). Importantly, there was a time-dependent response to the load – not only the current load, but also of past loads – and hence, the material could be said to have a memory of previous stresses.

Additionally, while elastic materials were shown to be able to store mechanical energy without dissipation of that energy, viscous (Newtonian) fluids were able to dissipate energy, without being able to store it. Clearly, what they were observing was a class of materials that not only had the capacity to both store and dissipate mechanical energy, but was also capable of time-dependent deformation under load. Such materials they referred to as *viscoelastic*.

The description of viscoelasticity has opened an entirely new window on the behaviour of biological materials and, in so doing, has emphasised time-dependent creep and recovery behaviour of structures such as joints, skin and blood vessels. It has also completely changed our view of synthetic fibres and polymeric materials.

As the name implies, viscoelasticity combines aspects of both viscosity (fluid behaviour) and elasticity (solid behaviour). While elastic materials store 100% of applied energy when they are deformed by an external force, viscoelastic materials lose or dissipate some energy under deformation. This loss or dissipation is known as hysteresis. Thus, the area between the loading and unloading curve of a viscoelastic material is the energy lost or hysteresis (Fig. 2.9a). The ability to dissipate energy is clearly a highly significant property of viscoelastic materials such skin, tendon and bone, because it gives them an inherent ability to absorb shock.

The other two main characteristics associated with viscoelastic materials are stress relaxation and creep. Stress relaxation is in some sense the inverse of creep, and refers to the general characteristic of viscoelastic materials to relax over time *under a fixed level of strain* (Fig. 2.9b). In contrast, creep refers to the ability of these materials to undergo increased deformation *under a constant stress* (Fig. 2.9c).

Viscoelastic materials such as skin, cartilage and jelly babies are characterised by the phenomenon of creep, which, as we have seen, is a time-dependent deformation under a constantly applied force. For instance, the stretching of skin under a constant load is due to collagen re-alignment, displacement of fluids, and fragmenting of elastic fibres. In addition to strong time dependence, creep is also dependent

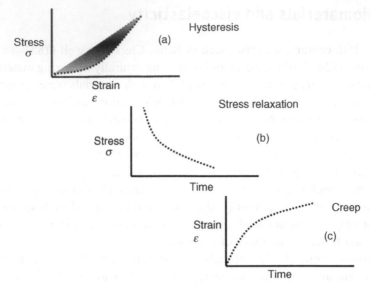

Figure 2.9 The behaviour of a viscoelastic material. (a) The area between the loading and unloading curve of a viscoelastic material (shaded) is the energy lost, or *hysteresis*. (b) *Stress relaxation*, which is the ability of viscoelastic materials to relax over time under a fixed level of strain. (c) *Creep*, or the ability to undergo increased deformation under a constant stress.

on temperature. Unlike metals, which are relatively stable over a broad range of ambient temperatures, viscoelastic materials experience quite radical changes in their response to stress and strain for moderate temperature changes. Time/temperature effects are based on the principle that they affect mainly the viscous nature of the material, with the primary effect of raising the temperature being to reduce the time scale of deformation. Decreased temperature lengthens the deformation time.

A final important concept is that viscoelastic materials can be distinguished from elastic materials by their memory of shape; whereas an elastic material only has the memory of its original shape, the deformation of a viscoelastic model is a function of the entire history of applied force (Terzopoulos and Fleischer, 1988).

The assumption of most mathematical constructs of viscoelasticity is that stress is proportional to strain at any given time, and such materials are referred to as being linearly viscoelastic. Unfortunately, in most biological materials stress and strain are not linearly related, with the key assumption of linearity for small strains only ($< 1\%$). Such substances are referred to as non-linear viscoelastic materials, and their behaviour is the subject of much ongoing research (Drapaca *et al.*, 2007). Since viscoelastic materials include cartilage, skin and bones, it is important to briefly look again at the viscous part of viscoelasticity. Viscosity in itself is not difficult to understand. It is simply defined as the ratio of the stress to strain rate; in other words, it is the ratio of the shear stress to the velocity gradient within a

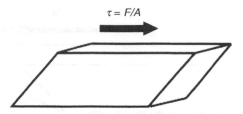

Figure 2.10 Shear of a body between a stationary surface and a force acting at a constant velocity parallel to the surface. The applied force per unit area of the plate is called the shear stress: $\tau = F/A$.

material when it starts to shear. To understand this, it is necessary to consider a form under shear (Fig. 2.10). The shear stress (τ, tau) is simply applied force divided by unit area: $\tau = F/A$.

Now consider a jelly baby being sheared between a stationary surface and your moving finger (Fig. 2.11). The top of the jelly baby moves at a constant velocity, v, by the action of the shearing force of your finger, F. Because the bottom of the jelly baby is stationary, different layers within the jelly baby move at different velocities. These differences in velocity cause a shearing action between layers, and the rate of shear (γ) is the relative displacement of one layer with respect to the next.

Let us return to Figure 2.10. As we now know, the shear force, F, divided by the contact area, A, gives the shear stress, τ. As we see in Figures 2.11 and 2.12, the shear rate, γ, is the difference in velocity between the layers. Because the bottom layer does not move, the shear rate can be calculated as the velocity of the top plate divided by the distance between the two ($\gamma = v/y$). The ratio of the shear stress and shear rate is the viscosity, η. Thick fluids such as honey have a high viscosity; thin

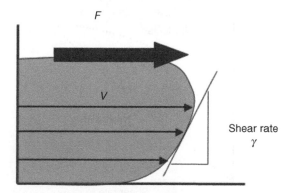

Figure 2.11 Consider a jelly baby being squashed with a shearing force F beneath a thumb moving at a constant velocity v. If the bottom of the jelly baby remains stationary, different layers within its substance will move at differing velocities, which causes friction (shearing action) between them. The rate of shear (γ) is the relative displacement of one layer with respect to the next and corresponds to the slope of the velocity profile.

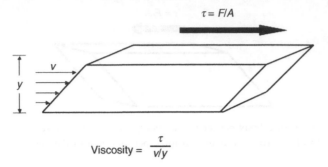

Figure 2.12 A body moving at a shear rate of $\gamma = v/y$ under an applied shear stress of τ. The applied force acts at a constant velocity parallel to the surface, and its magnitude per unit area is called the shear stress: $\tau = F/A$.

fluids such as water have a low viscosity. In other words, as the viscosity increases, it requires a larger force to move the top layers at a given velocity.

Intuitively, we understand the viscous behaviour of many of the fluids encountered in everyday life such as water and honey. These are described as being Newtonian. A Newtonian fluid is one in which the viscosity is independent of the shear rate. In other words, a plot of shear stress versus shear strain rate is linear in slope (Fig. 2.13). There are, however, many substances that do not follow Newtonian behaviour, such as egg white, blood or saliva. Such non-Newtonian liquids are distinguished by the fact that they have microscopic or molecular-level structures that can be rearranged substantially during flow. Think of the slipperiness of water between the fingers, and how it differs from that of blood. The slipperiness (viscosity) of non-Newtonian fluids changes a great deal depending on how fast they move or the forces applied to them. Other examples include the difference in how the surface of a fluid deforms when stirred; when you rotate a cylindrical rod

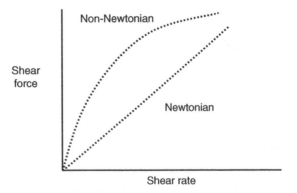

Figure 2.13 Schematic plot of shear force against shear strain rates for Newtonian and non-Newtonian fluids. Newtonian fluids have a linear relationship; in other words the viscosity is independent of shear rate. Non-Newtonian fluids have a non-linear relation, with viscosity decreasing at high shear rates. This is known as shear thinning.

inside a container of a Newtonian fluid, centrifugal forces cause the fluid to spread higher against the wall. For non-Newtonian fluids, the rotation results in the fluid climbing the rod; this is called the Weissenberg effect. As a Newtonian fluid leaves an opening, it tapers to a smaller cross-section, but the cross-section for a non-Newtonian fluid first increases before it eventually tapers. This phenomenon is called *die swell*.

Possibly the most striking behaviour of non-Newtonian fluids is a consequence of their viscoelasticity. Such substances have memory. If they are deformed through the action of a force, they return to their original shape when the force is removed. This happens when a rubber ball bounces; the ball is deformed as it hits a surface, but the rubber remembers its undeformed spherical shape. In contrast, Newtonian fluids have no memory; when a force is removed, they retain their condition at the time the force is removed. Non-Newtonian fluids are viscoelastic in the sense that they have a fading memory. While the fluid will remember its undeformed shape and return toward it, if the force is applied on the fluid for a long time, it will eventually forget its undeformed shape. If a sample of a non-Newtonian fluid is dropped onto a surface, it will bounce like a ball. However, if the fluid is simply placed on the surface, it will flow smoothly.

2.5 Acceleration and impact

Basically, impact is the striking of one body against another. It is important in forensics, simply because impacting objects with curved, angular or pointed surfaces can result in different types of soft tissue injury (see Chapter 4). According to the classic theory of impact, a body of mass m, moving with a velocity of v, has a momentum of mv. As Newton's second law showed, if a force F impacts on this body, there will be a change in momentum. This is of course only true if the two bodies cannot interpenetrate. And, according to Newton's third law, two impacting bodies have forces of action and reaction that are equal but opposite. This is clearly an oversimplification. Firstly, all elements within each impacting body are assumed to be rigidly connected and, hence, instantaneously subjected to the same altered motion as a result of the impact. However, we know that impact can result in the generation of longitudinal, transverse or torsional processes. Rigid body analysis is thus inadequate and must include consideration of the geometry and physical properties of the impacting bodies (Goldsmith, 2001). Furthermore, impacts can be either elastic (they conserve both momentum and kinetic energy) or plastic (they conserve momentum, but not kinetic energy). An example of elastic collision is a highly elastic ball dropped onto a concrete floor that bounces nearly to the height at which it was released. In a plastic (or inelastic) collision, the colliding objects stick together and, hence, travel at the same velocity. Thus, while velocities will change, total momentum will be conserved. A classic example of this is a motor vehicle colliding with a pedestrian. If it's a slow collision, the pedestrian will gently land on the bonnet to be carried away unhurt. However, if it happens at greater speed, the pedestrian will experience permanent and significant strain (probably fatal!). Such an irreversible deformation is of course the result of the conversion of kinetic energy into a permanent distortion of our pedestrian. Modelling of such a phenomenon can no longer be seen in Newtonian terms, but has to include two additional approaches: firstly, the hydrodynamic theory of impact and, secondly, the theory of plastic wave propagation (Goldsmith, 2001).

According to the hydrodynamic theory of impact, the medium under consideration is a compressible fluid through which shock waves can propagate. Alternatively, according to the theory of plastic strain propagation, the behaviour of the medium is described in terms of stress, strain and strain rate.

2.6 Fracture behaviour

For centuries, scientists have attempted to understand how structures fail, in the hope that this will lead to new designs better able to withstand the stresses and strains associated with their use. Our understanding of fracture mechanics has developed in fits and starts, with thousands of years of faltering progress from the first manufacture of primitive stone implements and tools until a major watershed was reached nearly a century ago, with the works of Charles Edward Inglis (1875–1952) and Alan Arnold Griffith (1893–1963). These two fathers of fracture mechanics presented a number of papers that finally established the concept of fracture energy and laid the groundwork of our present understanding of how structures fail under stress.

Engineers have known for a long time that neither strength nor stiffness is the most important factor in a given material, but that it is its toughness that is the critical property. In other words, the critical factor in fracture behaviour is the material's ability to resist the propagation of cracks within it (Gordon, 1991). Imagine an elastic material such as a simple rubber band. As the band is stretched, it stores more and more strain energy. Theoretically, there comes a point at which all of the chemical bonds within the band are stretched to their absolute maximum, after which it has to fail and release the energy stored. However, in practice, materials break much sooner than their predicted point of failure. In 1921, the 28-year-old engineer AA Griffith published a paper in the *Transactions of the Royal Society of London* in which he addressed this problem. Griffith showed the presence of numerous microscopic cracks in every substance, and believed that these flaws lowered the overall strength of the material. He then began to flesh out the relationship between the behaviour of a crack in terms of the energy involved in its propagation. Griffith's equation basically stated that, when a crack propagates through a material, the loss of strain energy is equal to the gain in surface energy. So, returning now to our example, the stretched elastic band will fail not at the point where the chemical bonds within it are stretched to their absolute maximum, but at a point of discontinuity somewhere along its length. The recognition that every material carries within it imperfections that may act as the sites of crack initiation raises two additional problems: firstly, once initiated, how do cracks progress? Secondly, once they start growing, how far will they progress? Answers to these questions rely heavily on Griffith's notion of the role of energy sources and sinks in crack propagation.

How does a crack progress? There are two ways of looking at it. The first is from the point of view of the stress intensity factor (SIF). Because the material resists cracking with everything it has, which is called its fracture toughness, the crack will only grow when its SIF becomes larger than the fracture toughness of the material.

Another way of looking at crack growth is by considering the energy lost during crack propagation. When a crack is formed, new surfaces are also formed along the edges where the material has split apart. Clearly, the material has to be subjected to enough energy to create these new surfaces or it will not crack.

How far will a crack progress? Things may change dramatically once a crack has grown. The resistance of the material may increase or decrease; the energy necessary to advance the fracture may also have gone up or down. In order for the crack to continue its progress, the change in energy must equal the change in resistance. If the change in energy is less than the change in resistance, then the crack will terminate unless more force is applied. If the change in energy is greater than the change in resistance, there will be unstable crack growth, in which case the crack may grow catastrophically until the entire structure fails.

Fractures may be classified according the process of fracture (the nature of the external forces applied to it) or according to the material properties itself.

Classification according to fracture process (Fig. 2.14)

Type I – forces acting perpendicular to the crack pull it open. An obvious example is a knife cut into skin or an axe chop into the head.

Type II – forces act parallel to the crack, with one force pushing the top half of the crack back and the other pulling the bottom half of the crack forward along the same line. The result is a shear fracture; in other words, the crack slides along itself. An example would be a compression fracture of a long bone.

Type III – forces pull in opposite directions, perpendicular to the crack. This results in the material separating out of its original plane. An example is tearing a sheet of paper.

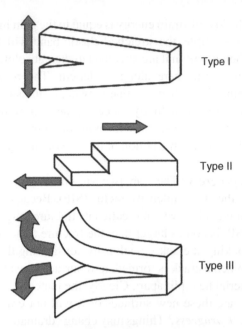

Figure 2.14 Classification of fractures according to process. Type I: forces acting perpendicular to the crack pull it open. Type II: forces act parallel to the crack, with one force pushing the top half of the crack back and the other pulling the bottom half of the crack forward along the same line. Type III: the forces pull in opposite directions, perpendicular to the crack. This results in the material separating out of its original plane.

Classification according to material properties

As we have seen, the fracturing process releases strain energy (internal potential energy of deformation) and, hence, for a fracture to propagate through a given material, the rate of energy released as the fracture grows has to be greater than a critical value.

Ductile fracture – for ductile materials such as steel, fracture is preceded by relatively slow deformation of the material, often associated with yielding or plastic flow, hence often associated with gross plastic deformation (Callister, 2003).

Brittle fracture – for brittle, low-toughness materials such as glass, fractures are usually sudden once the energy released by the fracture is equal to the energy required to create a free fracture surface. Hence, the critical stress for fracture is linearly related to the so-called stress intensity factor (SIF). In fracture mechanics the stress intensity factor, K, is used to predict the stress intensity or stress state near the tip of a crack caused by a remote load. When this stress state becomes critical, a small crack extends and the material fails. The load at which this failure occurs is referred to as the *fracture strength*. Importantly, minor flaws in the material can greatly influence the propagation of the crack (Sih, 1981). Often referred to as stress raisers, these flaws can amplify a stress at their locale, resulting in crack formation or propagation.

Viscoelastic fracture – the fracture process for viscoelastic materials such as skin and bone is more complex and less well understood. Not only does it have a time-dependent element, there is temperature dependence as well as a dependence on the stress/strain history. In fact, depending on the temperature and the rate of loading, viscoelastic materials can exhibit behaviours ranging from brittle fracture to viscous flow and, hence, they can be seen as a class of materials that form a transition between the ductile, rigid metals and the highly deformable liquids (Gross and Seelig, 2006).

2.7 Ballistic biomechanics

Thousands of scientific and not-so-scientific articles, chapters and books on ballistics have been written. This is a good thing, especially in view of the regrettable misconceptions that still exist regarding terminal ballistics and wounding potential. Popular writing is important here, as the massive amount of information in the scientific literature can be difficult to wade through, particularly for those who are averse to mathematical formulae. What is needed, particularly for those who are non-physicists, is a clear and accessible introduction to the subject, which is the purpose of this section.

The topic of ballistics has traditionally been subdivided into three general areas, each determined by what the projectile is doing. The science of what happens as the bullet accelerates down the barrel is termed *interior ballistics*, and the events that govern the movement of the bullet from the time it leaves the barrel to the time it strikes its target are referred to as *exterior ballistics*. The study of what happens from the moment of impact of the projectile is the field of *terminal (wound) ballistics*. Importantly, however, both interior and exterior ballistics, together with the design of the projectile, may have a profound effect on terminal ballistics. None of these factors will be discussed in this introductory section. Instead, we will highlight the basics of wound ballistics, with special attention to bone and skin wounding in the next two chapters. For a highly detailed account of the entire subject, the reader is referred to the superb text by Kneubuehl *et al.* (2011).

Kinetic energy at impact and wounding: kinetic energy is of vital importance when considering wounding, and is given by:

$$E = \frac{1}{2}m \cdot v^2$$

where E is the kinetic energy, m is the mass of the projectile, and v is its velocity.

As Kneubuehl and his co-authors have stressed, wounding only occurs when energy is transmitted to the target tissue. This they labelled E_{ab}. The relationship between the energy transmitted to the penetration distance, s, can thus be measured in joules per centimetre (Energy/Distance). The assumption that deceleration of the projectile in tissue is proportional to the square of its velocity allows for a wounding equation of:

$$E'_{ab} = -2 \cdot R \cdot E$$

where E'_{ab} is the wounding potential, R is what they termed the retardation coefficient and E the energy on impact.

Now we get to the important part of Kneubuehl's formula: R, the retardation coefficient, determines the energy transferred from the bullet to the tissue for a given distance. What this means is that bullets with the same impact energy, but with different values for R, transmit different magnitudes of energy to the tissue impacted. Alternatively, impact energy does not in itself dictate energy transferred for a given distance of penetration; rather, it is determined by the retardation coefficient times the impact energy. The question now is, of course, what exactly is R?

The retardation coefficient, R, is given as:

$$R = \frac{C_D \cdot \rho \cdot A}{2m}$$

where C_D is the drag factor of the projectile, which is shape dependent; ρ is the density of the tissue penetrated; A is the surface area of the projectile in contact with the tissue; and m is the mass.

Temporary cavitation of tissue: as the bullet passes through its target tissue, it creates a permanent shot channel, with roughly the same diameter as the bullet or its fragments. However, it also directs its kinetic energy to the walls of the shot channel, which violently drives the soft tissue away in a radial fashion. This results in a temporary cavity that has a diameter that is much larger than that of the projectile. Logically, the maximum diameter of the temporary cavity is only reached once the bullet has passed through the area. Within milliseconds, the temporary cavity collapses on itself and, depending on the elasticity of the tissues, may bounce back to form a second, smaller cavity. A number of short-term pulses of temporary cavitation may result. Hollerman *et al.* (1990) have stated that heavier, slower bullets crush more tissue, but result in smaller temporary cavitation when compared to lighter, faster bullets that leave a smaller shot channel, but result in a larger temporary cavity.

Theoretically, this leads to three zones of injury to soft tissues: firstly the central shot channel; secondly, a zone of vascular disruption; and finally, a stretch zone (Fig. 2.15).

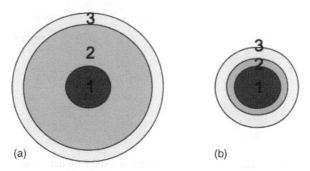

Figure 2.15 Idealised representation of the three zones of damage to soft tissue: 1, shot channel; 2, zone of vascular disruption; 3, stretch zone. Diagram (a) is at maximum temporary cavitation; (b) is after the bullet has passed through the target tissue.

Bullet factors in wounding: fragmentation and deformation are highly important bullet characteristics that are often deliberately manipulated to increase wounding. Originally, lead bullets tended to deform while jacketed rounds did not. Semi-jacketed or hollow-nosed bullets fragmented. Modern manufacturing techniques have lead to the ability to produce hollow-nosed bullets that in fact neither fragment nor deform. Of course, the target characteristics also have an important determining role to play. Whereas a fast, hollow-nosed bullet can pass though a thin layer of tissue without deformation, a thicker layer of the same tissue will require more time to penetrate and, hence, result in a visible change in shape. Whatever its cause, in semi-jacketed rounds, bullet deformation is rapid and is initiated at the exposed lead tip. Rifle bullets travel with substantially more energy than handgun bullets and, hence, because energy transfer is dependent on E'_{ab} (the wounding potential), rifle bullets generally cause larger shot channels than handgun bullets.

In addition to fragmentation and deformation, there is another important determinant of wounding that is directly related to how the projectile travels through the air, and that is the concept of *yaw*. The term *yaw* refers to any deviation of the longitudinal axis of the bullet from its line of flight; in other words, broadsiding. Yaw has a major effect on the bullet's impact profile, simply because the contact with the target is vastly increased (Fig. 2.16). It is thought that the tumbling moment of the projectile within the tissue also depends on the angle of impact (Kneubuehl *et al.*, 2011). A small angle of impact from a bullet travelling along a stable flight path will have a smaller tumbling moment than an unstable flight path characterised by yawing.

Wounding capacity: in summary, the actual wounding, or the efficiency of energy transfer between bullet and target tissue, depends on the following factors (Bartlett, 2003).

- The kinetic energy of the bullet.
- The impact profile of the bullet.

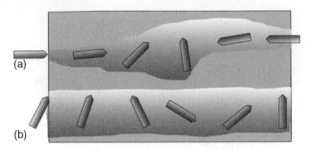

Figure 2.16 Schematic representation of tumbling of a stable bullet (a) through soft tissue, as opposed to a yawing bullet (b).

- Deformation or fragmentation of the bullet.

- The depth of penetration of the bullet.

- Biological characteristics of the target tissues.

- Temporary cavitation.

References

Bartlett CS. 2003. Clinical update: gunshot wound ballistics. *Clinical Orthopaedics and Related Research* **408**:28–57.

Callister WD. 2003. *Materials Science and Engineering*, 6th Edition. John Wiley & Sons, Inc., Hoboken, NJ.

Chailleux E, Davies P. 2003. A nonlinear viscoelastic viscoplastic model for behaviour of polyester fibres. *Mechanics of Time Dependent Materials* **9**:147–60.

Drapaca CS, Sivaloganathan S, Tenti G. 2007. Nonlinear constitutive laws in viscoelasticity. *Mathematics and Mechanics of Solids* **12**:475–501.

Goldsmith W. 2001. *Impact: The Theory and Physical Behaviour of Colliding Solids*. Dover Publications, New York.

Gordon JE. 1991. *The New Science of Strong Materials*. Penguin Books, London.

Griffith AA. 1921. The phenomena of rupture and flow in solids. *Philosophical Transactions of the Royal Society London A* **221**:163–98.

Gross D, Seelig T. 2006. *Fracture Mechanics*. Springer, Heidelberg.

Hollerman JJ, Fackler ML, Coldwell DM, Ben-Menachem Y. 1990. Gunshot wounds: 1. Bullets, ballistics and mechanisms of injury. *American Journal of Radiology* **155**:685–90.

Kneubuehl MP, Coupland RM, Rothchild MA, Thali MJ. 2011. *Wound Ballistics*. Springer, Berlin.

Markovitz H. 1977. Boltzmann and the beginnings of linear viscoelasticity. *Transactions of the Society of Rheology* **21**:381–98.

Sih GC. 1981. *Mechanics of Fracture*. Martinus Nijhoff, The Hague.

Sokolnikoff SI. 1983. *Mathematical Theory of Elasticity*, 2nd Edition. Krieger, Malabar, FL.

Terzopoulos D, Fleischer K. 1988. Modeling inelastic deformation: viscoelasticity, plasticity, fracture. *Computer Graphics* **22**:268–79.

3
Biomechanics of bone and bony trauma

Jules Kieser

3.1 Composition of bone

Bone is the lightweight, tough protective framework of the body. Bone also facilitates the production of blood in its marrow, provides a reservoir for calcium and phosphorus and facilitates sound transduction in our middle ear. It is a composite that consists mainly of organic material (Type I collagen 90%) and an impure version of calcium phosphate, known as hydroxyapatite (Currey, 2003). While collagen has good tensile strength, it performs poorly in compression. Hydroxyapatite, in contrast, has good compressive strength, but is a stiff, brittle material. Incredibly, bone can heal itself and remodel to resist stresses and strains. However, as we age, bone becomes more brittle, and this increases our susceptibility to injury.

Bone develops prenatally either from a cartilage or a membrane template. Ossification commences in around the fifth intra-uterine week and results in a relatively unorganised bone, called woven bone, which matures into cancellous or compact bone. Most weight-supporting bones (long bones) develop from a cartilage model which contains three ossification centres: the diaphysis, a central area that develops before birth, and two epiphyses – one at each end of the developing bone. Each of these contains a hyaline cartilage growth plate, from where bones continue to grow until skeletal maturity is reached. A trade-off takes place now. By giving up cartilage for mature bone, plasticity of cartilage is sacrificed for the rigidity imposed by mineralisation. The implications for trauma are discussed later. Bones of the face are formed by the direct transformation of connective tissue into bone by bone-forming cells, called osteoblasts (for review, see Meikle, 2002).

Osteoblasts are extremely important for the formation and maintenance of bone. Burgess and Maciag (1989) were among the first to distinguish between their role of promoting mineralisation of the organic matrix and their function as synthesisers of extracelullar growth factors. Bone is made up of mineral salts in the form of calcium phosphate and calcium hydroxide that form hydroxyapatite crystals, given as $Ca_{10}(PO_4)_6(OH)_2$. Some of these form covalent bonds with long strands of Type I collagen. As the bone ossifies, cells (called osteocytes) become incorporated into the matrix, where they exist in tiny spaces called lacunae, which are inter-connected by slender canals, or canaliculi, through which they communicate and receive oxygen and nutrients. Osteocytes, imprisoned in their lacunae, are arranged in a radial fashion around a central canal, thus forming an osteon or Haversian

Forensic Biomechanics, First Edition. Jules Kieser, Michael Taylor and Debra Carr.
© 2013 John Wiley & Sons, Ltd. Published 2013 by John Wiley & Sons, Ltd.

system. Osteons, in turn, are arranged along the long axis of the bone, where they are surrounded by concentric layers of bone called lamellae, giving the impression of layers of plywood that strengthen and protect the inner parts of the bone.

Significantly, bone is a dynamic system that continuously renews and restructures itself. The importance of mechanical loading to the determination of the structure and remodelling of all the bones in the body is traditionally attributed to Julius Wolff (1836–1902). He and others suggested that bony trabeculae are laid down along lines of maximal compressive and tensile stress, referred to as stress trajectories. What this means, in effect, is that the structure of a bone is morphologically adapted to its function in line with biomechanical principles – the so-called Wolff's law. Of course, it is important to remember that bones not only adapt as a result of daily activity, but also that the skeleton is evolutionarily adapted to its function.

3.2　Types of bone

Bone can conveniently be divided into two types: cortical (compact) and cancellous (trabecular) bone (Fig. 3.1). The ends of long bones, such as the humerus, have an outer shell of cortical bone with a spongy, cancellous inner core. Flat bones, such as those of the scapula or the cranium, have the same setup, but with a thin central cancellous layer sandwiched between two dense cortical outer layers. At the microscopic level, bone consists of sheets of mineralised collagen fibres often wrapped around a central canal to form the Haversian systems (or osteons) referred

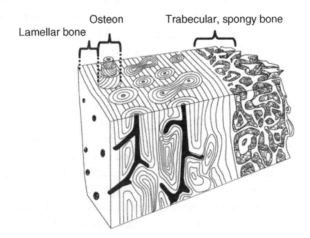

Figure 3.1　The structure of bone. Lamellae encircle the periphery of the bone. Concentric lamellae arranged around a central vascular channel are called osteons or Haversian systems. In longitudinal section, vascular channels are shown to interconnect with adjacent osteons as well as the outer surface of the bone. Trabecular or spongy bone forms the inner layer.

to above. On the outside, lamellae are stacked like plywood around the entire circumference of the bone, called lamellar bone.

The composition and structure of both compact and cancellous bone vary with factors such as age, anatomical site, sex, physiological function and, of course, its regular loading pattern. These factors, when combined with its structural design, make bone highly heterogeneous indeed. This of course means that even a 'typical' bone is so complex that one cannot recognise a single level of organisation that is characteristic of it. For instance, it is misleading to think of cancellous bone as being compact bone with holes in it. Although its *tissue* is made up of bony elements, its design of struts and trabeculae gives it a unique *material* behaviour. Traditionally, scientists have subscribed to the belief that trabeculae are arranged in relation to the principal stresses in bone (Wolff's law) and, hence, that cancellous bone is designed to absorb energy. Debate continues about the role of cancellous bone during biomechanical loading, but what we do know is that trabeculae are not homogeneous and, hence, the distribution of stresses within it is difficult to determine (Currey, 2002).

3.3 Biomechanical properties of bone

Bone strength is influenced by anatomical factors such as size, shape and architecture, and also by physiological properties such as bone quality and bone mineral density. One of the major functions of bone is to carry loads (the other is blood production). Clearly, when these loads exceed the bone strength, fracturing will result. We can define bone strength by a number of biomechanical parameters, including its strength (ultimate force), toughness, brittleness, stiffness and work to failure. As a young bone matures, it becomes more mineralised. Increased mineralisation improves the structural rigidity of bone, but at the same time makes it more brittle (Currey, 1969). Healthy adult bones must therefore have an optimal combination of stiffness and brittleness; while young, poorly mineralised bone tends to be weak, old hypermineralised bone is brittle (Fig. 3.2).

A controversial issue is the strength of bone. Whichever way one looks at it, there are two sides to the issue: firstly, a *material side* that looks at stiffness and ductility and their relationship to the elastic modulus as well as other useful measures such as the Poisson ratio, work to fracture, yield strength and so on. The other side of the coin is the *structural perspective*, which looks at the size and shape of the bone in relation to its strength. By doing this, we can explore how regional or local variations in architecture influence the stiffness or toughness of bone. If bony tissue were uniform in its composition and shape, every bone would fail at the same stress, irrespective of whether it is a humerus, a femur or a rib. Moreover, in the past decade scientists have emphasised the hierarchical structure of bone, particularly at

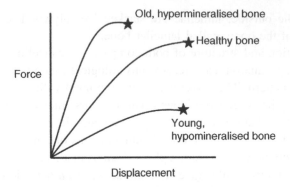

Figure 3.2 Healthy bone has an optimum balance between stiffness and ductility. Old bone is hypermineralised, hence brittle. Young bone is hypomineralised and can thus deform considerably before fracture.

the micro- and nanostructural levels, and how this relates to its biomechanical properties. What they showed was that scale was critically important and, hence, different techniques had to be used to investigate material properties at the different size levels. Figure 3.3 illustrates these, included in which are the macrostructural levels of cortical and cancellous bone (a), the microstructural levels of osteons, Haversian systems and trabeculae (b), the sub-microstructural level of lamellae

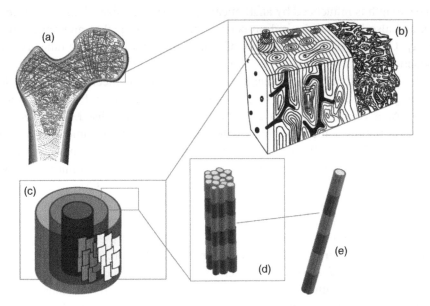

Figure 3.3 The importance of scale in bone architecture. (a) Macrostructure of cancellous and cortical bone; (b) microstructural scale of osteons, Haversian systems and trabeculae; (c) sub-microscopic scale of lamellae; (d) nanostructure of collagen fibres; (e) sub-nanoscale of individual collagen fibrils and embedded mineral. (Adapted from Rho *et al.*, 1989.)

(c), the nanoscale level of collagen bundles (d) and, finally, the sub-nanoscale level of individual fibrils and bone crystals (e). We will deal with each of these sequentially to see how they influence the biomechanical properties of bone.

Macrostructural level: as we have seen, bone can be divided into compact (cortical) bone and cancellous (trabecular) bone (Fig. 3.1). Cortical bone is essentially solid, with enough porosity to accommodate the occasional cells and vascular channels. It makes up the dense outer surface of all bones. Cancellous bone is spongy and fills the inside of many bones. The best way of visualising the mechanical properties of cortical bone is to look at a typical stress/strain curve for such bone loaded in tension (Fig. 3.4). Notice that the graph has two major parts: first it has a straight path up to the yield point, followed by a flat part until the bone fails. In the first part, bone behaves in a linear elastic fashion; in other words, when the force is removed it will return to its original dimensions, and the lengthening will be directly proportional to the force magnitude. The slope of this part of the curve gives Young's modulus of elasticity, which is a measure of the stiffness (as we have seen before). The area beneath the curve, called its resilience, is the amount of energy that the bone can absorb without permanent deformation. This is the elastic field.

Once the curve flattens out, bone behaves viscoelastically in that it yields, and the bone becomes more or less permanently deformed (plastic deformation). Increasing the tensile force results in further lengthening of the bone, with deformation persisting after the force is removed. The area under the curve is a measure of how much work is required before the bone fails completely; this is the plastic field. Clearly, a brittle bone will experience very little deformation whereas a tough bone will show a great deal of deformation before it breaks.

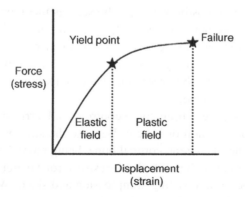

Figure 3.4 Biomechanical properties of compact bone as illustrated by a force-displacement curve loaded in tension. The slope of the curve up to the yield point is the Young's modulus of elasticity (a measure of the stiffness). Between the yield point and failure, the bone behaves viscoelastically.

Of course, bone does not break with the appearance of the first crack. In fact its design allows it to mount a rear-guard action against the spread of cracks, and it can do this at all levels of its construction. This resistance to fracture becomes more and more critical as one approaches the point of failure, and, hence, attention has focused on what happens after the yield point has been reached. But researchers are only now starting to understand the biomechanics of plastic deformation in bone. Although individual processes have been identified, an integrated model of plastic deformation is extremely complicated and imperfectly understood even today. We will return to this issue a little later.

There are two special properties of bone that we have to consider before we deal with fracture behaviour. The first is the fact that the biomechanical behaviour of bone does not only depend on the magnitude of the applied force, but also on its direction and rate of application (Cullinane and Einhorn, 2002). Whereas ideal materials are *isotropic* – in other words, they behave in the same fashion regardless of loading direction – bone is *anisotropic*, because its mechanical properties differ under different loading directions. So, for instance, the strength and rigidity of the femur is greater under compression (its customary loading during walking or jumping), than when a load is applied in a transverse direction.

The second special feature of bone is its viscoelastic behaviour: if you apply force to bone and hold it at a constant strain, you find that the stress needed to hold it decreases. In other words, if a bone is loaded and kept there, it undergoes strain deformation – it 'creeps'. This of course means that bone loaded slowly has a different Young's modulus than bone loaded rapidly. Under low strain rates, bone flows like a viscous liquid, while the same bone behaves like a brittle elastic solid when subjected to a high strain rate such as blunt or ballistic trauma (Einhorn, 1992).

In contrast to cortical bone, cancellous bone consists of an interconnected network of rods, visible to the naked eye. The space between these struts is filled with marrow, and, being mostly water, can be seen as incompressible. The microarchitecture of cancellous bone makes it extremely difficult to characterise. Situated at the end of long bones and in the spinal column, cancellous bone fills all of the inner vertebral space. In the long bones it directs loads from the joints onto the midshaft of the bone; in lumbar vertebrae, cancellous bone carries and transfers about 90% of the applied load.

Now we have to enter the entirely more controversial territory of what happens if bone is loaded in compression or is bent. Because the stiffness of bone is largely determined by its mineral content, cortical bone, being more dense than cancellous bone, is hard and brittle, which means that it resists torque better than the cancellous bone. The latter is better at resisting compression and shear. What we do know is that the Young's modulus of cancellous bone is a function of its apparent trabecular density. When bone is compressed it is squashed down on itself and it can fail in a direction that is different from the direction of the load. Bending is even more complex than compression because the strain generated is different at different levels of the bone. Often the bone holds together, even though the load has gone past the yield point (Currey, 2003).

Microstructural level: evidence from a number of laboratories is mounting that, during loading, there is a significant positive relationship between local micro-architecture and microdamage to trabecular bone (Nagaraja *et al.*, 2005; Fratzl, 2008). What is also emerging is that microdamage actually begins at strains lower than the yield point of the bone. These microcracks accumulate during repetitive force, and are the bone's way of dissipating the energy impacted upon it. Because these microcracks can easily heal by remodelling, they are a very useful way of increasing the toughness of bone. Microcracks in the cortical bone tend to follow longitudinal cement lines, where osteons meet (Koester *et al.*, 2008). To withstand fracture, bone has to dissipate the elastically stored energy from an applied force. Because the propagation of a crack requires energy, the more energy dissipation mechanisms a material has, the tougher it will be. Microcrack propagation is one such mechanism, but there are other, more subtle ways in which bone resists breaking, and these operate at a smaller level.

Nanoscale level: at the smallest level, bone consists of soft collagen strands that give it its elasticity and the ability to dissipate energy under mechanical deformation. Individual collagen fibrils deform by stretching and unwinding, which enables bone to withstand large strains before catastrophically fracturing. But there are two other mechanisms operating here that we are only just starting to understand: the role of mineral in stiffening bone and the concept of sacrificial bonds. What we know is that the collagen bundles in bone are interspersed by mineral platelets (Fig. 3.5). Continuous slip between collagen bundles is dampened by the mineral/ collagen interfaces between fibres (Ritchie, 2010). Additionally, the toughness of bone is augmented by tiny fibrils between collagen fibres, held together by hydrogen bonds. These act as a reversible glue that holds the structure together. In other words, energy is dissipated by breaking them, and, hence, they are referred to as 'sacrificial bonds' (Nalla *et al.*, 2003).

Toughness of bone: as we have seen, bone biomechanics is now considered from a hierarchical perspective. This is an incredible advance because it showed for the first time the different levels at which bone is adapted to withstand the normal (and some abnormal) forces applied to it. To do this, bone has to be tough. How does it work? The answer to this question again lies in considering different scales or levels of operation. The advance of a fracture through a substance, such as bone, has been likened to a competition between those mechanisms that facilitate crack growth ahead of the fracture path, and those mechanisms that inhibit it (Ritchie, 1999; Launey *et al.*, 2010). The first such toughening measure is that of crack deflection (Fig. 3.6a). Here the progression of a crack is influenced by its relation to gross morphological features such as the osteons. As the crack progresses, it is deflected at points of weakness around the osteons, thus slowing it down.

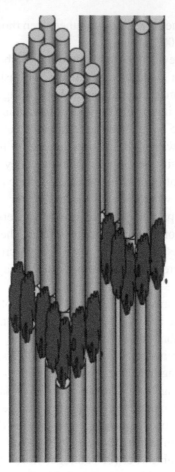

Figure 3.5 Schematic representation of columns of collagen fibres and their interspersed mineral crystals. (Adapted from Rho *et al.*, 1998.)

The next level at which bone enhances its toughness is that of constrained microfracture around the crack tip (Fig. 3.6b). Bone has a natural ability to develop, and then repair, microcracks. These tiny cracks are thought to dilate the area around the fracture tip, thus compressing the crack tip and slowing its progression (Ritchie, 1999). The third mechanism relies on the formation of smaller cracks ahead of the advancing crack tip (Fig. 3.6c). The uncracked bits of bone absorb energy and, hence, also slow down the process of fracturing. Finally, unbroken collagen fibrils that bridge the fracture increase toughness by resisting crack progression (Fig. 3.6d).

A final note on bone toughness. Bone is anisotropic and, hence, all of these toughening strategies are dependent on the orientation of the direction of the crack. Cracks propagate faster along the long axis of a bone than perpendicular to it. Slitting a bone is thus easier than breaking it.

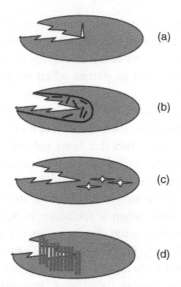

Figure 3.6 Schematic representation of the toughening mechanisms of bone. (a) Crack deflection where a crack deviates radically from its path; (b) formation of microcracks near the main fracture line; (c) crack-tip driving force is dissipated by secondary cracks forming ahead of fracture; (d) collagen fibrils bridge the fracture, thus dissipating fracture energy by sacrificial bonds. (Adapted from Peterlink *et al.*, 2006.)

3.4 Compressive and tensile fracture patterns

Recall that when a force is applied to a given bone it will experience an inner resistance to that force; this stress will be equal in magnitude, but opposite in direction to the applied force. Stress is expressed as force per unit area and measured in Pascals. Under the influence of the stress, the bone will change its dimensions – described as strain. Although bones are usually subjected to complex forces, these can be resolved into three basic types: *compression*, resulting from two opposite forces acting along the same line; *tension*, resulting from two opposing forces directed away from one another along the same line; and *shear*, resulting from two opposing forces acting parallel to one another, but not along the same line.

As we have seen in the previous chapter, when an elongated structure, such as a long bone, is loaded perpendicular to its long axis, it bends. The outer, convex surface experiences tensile stress, and the inner, concave surface experiences compressive stress. While tensile and compressive stresses are at a maximum on the outer surfaces of the bone, its centre experiences no stress. A serious weakness in this sort of reasoning, of course, is that long bones are not usually subjected to bending only. For instance, torsion results when a bone experiences a torque or twisting force. Torsion results in shear stresses along the shaft of the bone that can result in spiral fractures.

Obviously, in real life bone is not subjected purely to the simple types of force described above. Forces are applied to bone in a manifold manner that may include both axial and oblique angles and result in highly complex stress relationships. Bones show different mechanical properties when subjected to forces applied in different directions; a property known as *anisotropy*. Anisotropy is under the influence of the microarchitecture of cancellous bone that results in preferential oriented strength paths within the bone itself (Sugita *et al.*, 1999).

Currey (1999) highlighted the fact that bone behaves differently under tension compared to how it behaves when bent. When loaded in tension, bone shows a sharply defined yield region that is absent when it is loaded under bending (Fig. 3.7). While bending strength appears to be simple to measure, its simplicity may in fact be misleading. As we have seen, when a specimen is bent, one side is loaded in compression and the other in tension. Strain varies (in theory anyway), with the distance from the neutral axis. There is another factor at work here, originally introduced by Weibull (1951). He argued that a specimen under tension undergoes roughly the same stress all through its volume. In contrast, a bending specimen undergoes high tensile stresses only within a rather small volume on the surface opposite the point of loading. Bone is clearly not uniform and, hence, has a distribution of strengths throughout its volume. It is likely, Weibull stated, that a specimen in tension will yield at a lower calculated stress than a bending specimen, simply because the stress in a tensile specimen has a larger volume and thus, logically, more chance of incorporating a weaker area. The end result is that the outer fibres on the convex surface of a bent specimen fail earlier than a specimen loaded in tension.

When we think of stresses that develop in biological structures, we need to think in terms of how loads are applied to them. Hence, a long bone can be visualised as a beam when it is bent, a column when it is axially compressed and a shaft when it

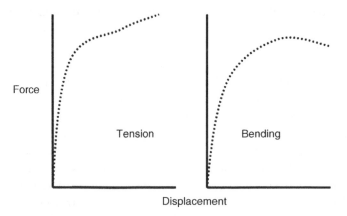

Figure 3.7   Compact bone behaves differently when loaded in tension as opposed to bending. Under tension there is a sharply defined yield point that is absent during three-point bending. (Adapted from Currey, 1999.)

experiences torsion. Moreover, a long bone is always supported at least at one end and free at the other, in which case it acts like a cantilevered beam. When it is attached at both ends (such as a femur when one is standing), it acts as a fixed column. Finally, one has to consider the biomechanics of bones subjected to both static and dynamic loads. The former are of long duration, with little change in force, magnitude or direction of application. In contrast, dynamic loads are variable in timing, magnitude and direction. This information now needs to be applied to our understanding of how shape and size influence the relative magnitudes of stresses that develop in bones during loading. Engineers use the concept of *moment of area*, together with the *material modulus of elasticity* in their mathematical descriptions of the failure of materials such as bone.

We now return to the question of how strong bone is. Here we deal with idealised compact bone and disregard its shape. In the next section we will focus on how real bone can withstand blunt and sharp forces and, if they can't, how they break.

There are a number of ways of looking at bony fracture:

- *Yield strength* is the highest stress developed in the bone before it shows plastic deformation (Fig. 3.8a).

- *Fracture strength* is the stress developed in bone at its point for fracture (Fig. 3.8b).

- *Ultimate strength* is the highest stress developed in bone before failure (Fig. 3.8c).

- *Impact strength* is a measure of a bone's ability to withstand shock loading.

- *Fatigue strength* is the magnitude of fluctuating or repetitive stress that a bone can experience before failing.

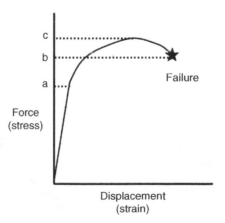

Figure 3.8 An idealised stress/strain curve for bone, illustrating the yield strength (a) which is the highest stress developed in the bone before it shows plastic deformation; the fracture strength (b), which is the stress developed in bone at its point for fracture; and the ultimate strength (c), which is the highest stress developed in bone before failure.

In answer to the question 'how strong is a given bone?' we have to think both in terms of what the bone is made of (i.e. the material properties such as its modulus), and its size and shape. While size and material properties are important determinants of strength, there is a third factor to consider. This is *second moment of area*, which relates to the bone's shape. Hence, it is not only the material that the bone is made of, nor its cross-sectional area that is important, but the shape of its cross-sectional area as well. The second moment of area of a bone is a geometrical property that depends on a reference axis. The smallest moment of area about an axis passes through the centroid of the bone, which is also called the *first moment of area*. The product of the elastic modulus and the second moment of area measures the ability of a bone to resist bending – called flexural stiffness. An I-shaped beam clearly has a higher resistance to bending than a rod-shaped beam, because it has a higher second moment of area. However, I-beams are not as strong as rods in torsion. Twisting via an applied torque is best resisted by pipe-like structures such as long bones. The ability to withstand twisting or torque is measured by the *polar area moment*.

To understand the foregoing better, consider a random bone, such as a humerus. If you suspend it from a string, the line of action will always pass through the centre of gravity or centroid of the bone. Since it is a three-dimensional object, the centroid can be determined by tying the string a number of times and noting the line of action of the string each time (Fig. 3.9). The point of intersection of these lines corresponds to the centroid – the point within a bone from which the force of gravity appears to act. This is the first moment of area. The second moment of area describes the capacity of an object's (in this case the bone's) cross-section to withstand bending.

The importance of the second moment of area (aka second moment of inertia) is immediately obvious when one considers two planks of equal dimensions loaded in

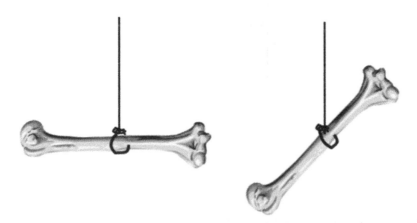

Figure 3.9   The centroid of a three-dimensional object can be visualised by suspending it at different angles; the point of intersection of the lines of action describes a point within the object from which gravity appears to act.

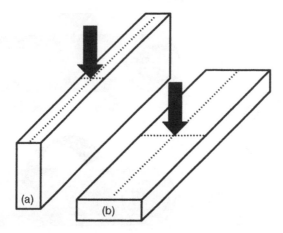

Figure 3.10 Schematic representation illustrating the effect of shape on stiffness of two beams with similar dimensions.

exactly the same fashion (Fig. 3.10). Intuitively, we know that the end-on loaded plank (a) will be stiffer than the other (b). The same is true for other shapes, such as I, L and H bars, as well as tubes, such as long bones.

As we saw in the previous chapter, bending of a long structure such as a beam or a long bone results in compressive stresses on the concave side and tensile stresses on the convex side (Fig. 3.11). Because bone is stronger in compression than in tension, it usually fractures on the tensile side first. Long bones are essentially tubular structures, whose moments of area can be calculated as follows (Fig. 3.12); the second moment of area is given as:

$$I = [\Pi(r_o^4 - r_i^4)]/4$$

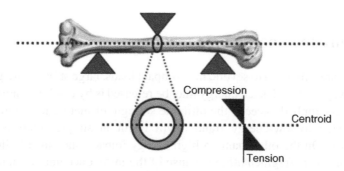

Figure 3.11 Bending a long bone results in both tensile and compressive stresses, the magnitudes of which are greatest at the surface of the bone and zero at the neutral axis (centroid). (Adapted from Turner and Burr, 1993.)

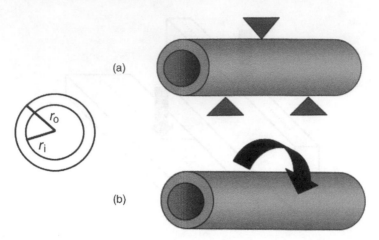

Figure 3.12 (a) The second moment of area in a tube subjected to bending; and (b) the polar moment of area in a tube subjected to torque (r_o = outer radius, r_i = inner radius of the cylinder).

and the polar moment of area as:

$$J = [\Pi(r_o^4 - r_i^4)]/2$$

What this means of course, is that bone strength is determined by a larger outer radius, rather than bone wall thickness.

There is another factor that influences the stiffness and strength of a bone. For a given cross-sectional area, the longer the bone, the larger the magnitude of stress produced at the point of application. Because of their length, long bones in humans and larger animals are subjected to high bending moments. In other words, they are constantly being subjected to high tensile, compressive and torsional stresses. Their tubular shape, together with their unique hierarchical structure, gives our bones the ability to withstand all of these complex bending moments.

3.5　Blunt and sharp force trauma

When bones are subjected to severe, high-impact loads, large stresses are generated. One of the ways in which such energy may be released is by crack initiation. Hence, once the stress applied exceeds the ultimate strength of that bone, it will fracture. Bone subjected to low-energy trauma will result in simple fractures, without fragmentation. On the other hand, a high-energy impact, such as a bullet wound, will result in severe fragmentation because of the instant accumulation of massive levels of energy released (Turner, 2006).

Bony trauma is a leading cause of morbidity across the globe. Accidents, disasters, assaults, sport and disease all contribute to this phenomenon.

Case 3.1 Postmortem and perimortem blunt force injury

Skeletal trauma analysis can offer critical data in a death investigation. The identification, patterning and interpretation of injuries to the skull often provide information that may have been lost as a result of soft tissue decomposition. Dry bones, such as those in (a), have a much-reduced moisture content. Hence, the fractured edges tend to be irregular and blunt. Additionally, the edges tend to be lighter in colour than those of the surrounding bone, as they are exposed to the environment at a later stage – in other words, after decomposition.

In fresh bones such as those in (b), the curvature of the skull at the point of impact tends to flatten out, and, as a result, the force of the impact is distributed over a relatively larger area. The bone surrounding the area of impact may then experience secondary and tertiary fractures that include linear or radiating fractures and curvilinear concentric fractures. Radiating fractures tend to terminate in concentric fractures, resulting in a typical spider-web appearance.

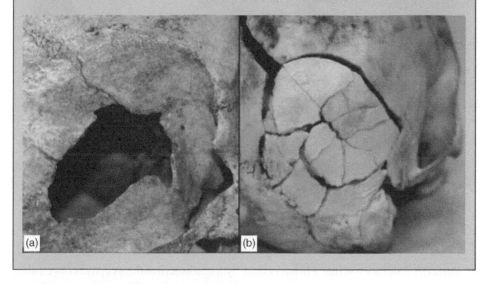

Classification of such fractures depends on one's profession. Orthopaedic, paediatric or maxillofacial surgeons have different classifications of bony trauma to those of pathologists or forensic anthropologists. Fractures can be classified according to morphology, to anatomical location or to causation. While we will not attempt to fully classify bony trauma, we do have to recognise some basic fracture types, and relate these to the biomechanics of bone. At the most basic level, a fracture can be *open* (exposed) or *closed* (covered by skin); and *complete* (fracture ends separated) or *incomplete* (fragments partially joined).

Case 3.2   Sharp force injury to the skull

Machete attacks are relatively common in agricultural areas of developing countries. Specifically, such attacks played a large role in the Rwandan massacres of Tutsis in 1994. These implements, used for routine bush clearing, have no legal restrictions on their possession. In the first case (a), from South Africa, a single cut has resulted in a well-marked incision on the side of the skull. In the second case (b), also from South Africa, three machete cuts have resulted in long, wedge-shaped incisions on the back of the skull. Note the consistency of wound patterning between the two cases.

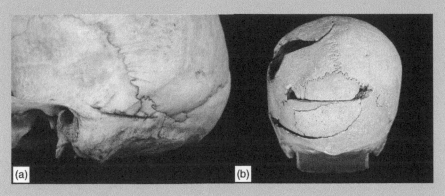

(Photos: M. Steyn)

Biomechanically, the following fracture types of long bones are recognised (Fig. 3.13):

- *Simple fracture* – results from relatively low-energy impact.

- *Comminuted fracture* – results from a high-energy impact.

- *Butterfly fracture* – when a bone is bent by a unidirectional force, the convex side undergoes tension and the concave side compression. Shear fracture planes, running at 45° to the surface of the bone, can result in the creation of a triangular fragment, resembling a butterfly.

- *Spiral fracture* – results from torsional or rotational forces applied to a long bone, such as violent turning of the foot, resulting in a spiral fracture of the tibia.

- *Buckled fracture* – occurs when a long bone is subjected to compression, unevenly applied. Here the force acts slightly off-centre, or the bone has a natural curvature and the compressive side of the bone buckles.

- *Greenstick fracture* – occurs due to compression or unidirectional force applied to young bone, which fractures much like a green branch. The outer cortex fractures, while the inner cortex bends.

- *Stellate fracture* – results from a high-energy impact to flat bones such as those of the skull.

- *Depressed fracture* – can result from a direct impact to a flat bone, such as a hammer blow, resulting in a sharply punched out wound created by shearing forces.

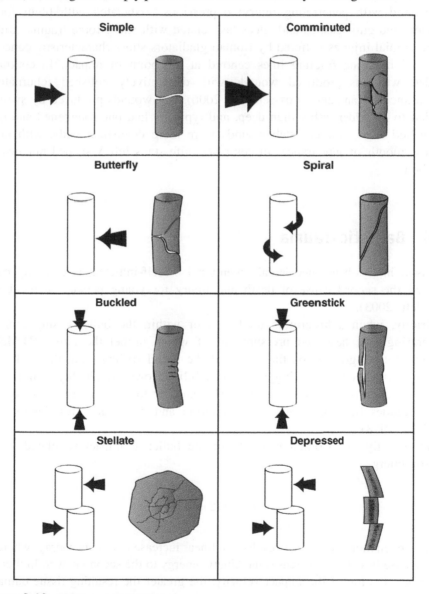

Figure 3.13 Fracture modes in bone.

Lovell (1997) has drawn attention to the difficulties in interpreting bony fracture patterns. She suggested that, despite the fact that fracture type can be related to proximate cause (as we have done in Fig. 3.13), the interpretation of the ultimate cause may be much more difficult. For instance, a fracture of a long bone in an older female might be secondary to osteoporosis rather than direct trauma. The principal aim of most classificatory protocols, however, remains to establish standardised descriptions related to injury mechanisms. One such method is that of Filer (1992), who categorised cranial injuries into piercings, associated with penetrating injury; depressions, associated with blunt force impact; and cuts, gashes and slices, associated with sharp force trauma. Blunt force cranial injuries suffered by Roman gladiators show characteristic concentric and radiating fracture lines centred at the point of impact. In contrast, bladed weapons produced wounds with distinctively polished (eburnated) appearances (Kanz and Grossschmidt, 2006). Cut wounds produced by swords tended to be wider rather than deep, and typically had one roughened and one burnished edge, whereas stab wounds were more deep than wide, with both edges smooth in appearance. In contrast, knife stabs left V-shaped notches in the bone.

3.6   Ballistic trauma

Ballistic injury, being accidental, intentional or self-inflicted, is currently considered the second cause of death and injury for young persons in the USA (Bartlett, 2003).

Briefly, when a firearm is fired, primer within the bullet casing ignites, generating gas, heat and pressure, all of which propel the bullet (DiMaio, 1998). Helical grooves on the inside of the barrel (rifling) spin the bullet on its long axis, hence giving it gyroscopic stability. However, a highly complex set of forces operating on the bullet in flight causes it to rotate in a rosette pattern that includes both the concepts of nutation and precession (for details, see DiMaio, 1998).

Importantly, the wounding ability of the bullet at impact is related to its kinetic energy,

$$E = 1/2\,m \cdot v^2$$

Hence, an increase in mass results in a linear increase in kinetic energy; whereas an increase in velocity increases the kinetic energy to the second power. In theory, therefore, the higher the impact velocity, the greater the resulting tissue damage

(Ming *et al.*, 1988). More realistically, Bartlett (2003) lists seven factors that determine the degree of disruption caused by ballistic impact:

1. kinetic energy at impact;

2. projectile movement;

3. calibre, shape and construction of the projectile;

4. the distance travelled through soft tissue;

5. biomechanical properties of the biological tissues penetrated;

Case 3.3   Blunt force versus ballistic injury

Impacts that transfer energy to bodily tissues can cause bony fracture, the pattern and extent of which will depend on the rate of energy deposition. Severe long bone fracture may arise from high local energy transfer, and may be due either to instantaneous transfer of energy, or its concentration on a small area. The way in which the energy is transferred therefore affects the break: a long bone fracture, caused by a blunt force impact with low- to medium-energy transfer may present as a clear breach; whereas a highly comminuted fracture will result from the virtual instantaneous transfer of massive energy to a small area. Figure (a) illustrates this concept; a clear humeral fracture was the result of blunt force trauma involving a motor vehicle. Figure (b) shows the shattered long bone in a sheep shot with a .22 long rifle.

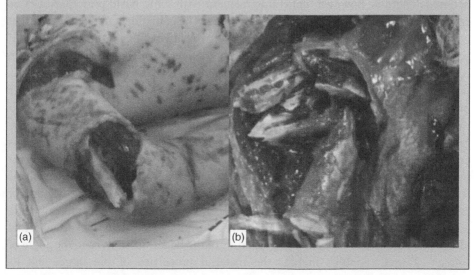

Case 3.4   Execution or suicide?

This photograph illustrates two types of bullet wounds to the back of the head. On the left is a typically well-defined entrance wound, which is the result of a single gunshot to the back of the head, execution style. On the right is the funnel-shaped exit wound on the back of the head of a suicide victim who had shot himself in the mouth.

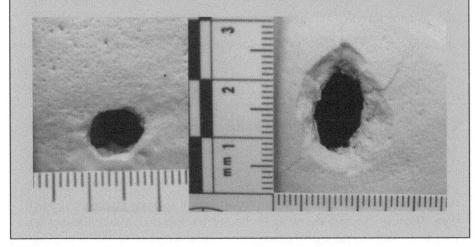

6. primary and secondary cavitation;

7. bullet fragmentation.

The issue of the biomechanics of ballistic bony trauma is controversial and much debated. There is, however, general agreement with some basic principles. Let us consider a bullet that impacts a thick, hard bone. The collision generates a force that will compress the bone and, if the impact energy is large enough, the projectile will penetrate the bone to continue its trajectory. Of course, the bone generates an opposing force on the bullet tip, which may result in its deformation or fracture. As we saw earlier, the impact may be analysed in terms of the overall energy of the projectile. In the instant before impact, the bullet has a kinetic energy equal to half the mass of the bullet, m, multiplied by the square of its velocity v^2. Suppose the bullet penetrates into the substance of the bone and then stops. Because energy is conserved, pre-impact kinetic energy is converted into inelastic deformation of bullet and bone, heat and sound. The work done by the bullet to penetrate the bone is related to the force of impact, times the depth of penetration. Obviously, whether or not the bullet passes through the bone will depend on whether the pre-impact kinetic energy is sufficient to drive it through the target. Among the projectile variables that affect this process are the material properties of the bullet, its shape and the angle of impact. Target variables include the material properties of the target and its thickness. Finally, there is another factor to bear in mind when considering the damage caused by ballistic impact: that of the momentum transfer. When a bullet strikes its target, there is an instant transfer of momentum, simply because, as the bullet hits the target, the target exerts an equal but opposite force on the bullet.

Before considering bony wounding, let us define some very basic concepts. Firstly, the entrance of a ballistic missile into a target, without completion of its passage through it, is referred to as *penetration*, which usually results in crater formation with embedment of the projectile. Secondly, the bullet can *rebound or ricochet* off the impacted surface and follow an altered trajectory, at reduced velocity. Finally, it can *perforate*, in which case the target is completely breached. Importantly, each of these processes occurs at miniscule time frames of several hundred milliseconds or less (Backman and Goldsmith, 1978).

From a theoretical point of view, depending on the thickness of the target tissue, a non-perforating impact (where plastic deformation exceeds hydrodynamic stresses in a relatively thin target), results in dishing or in-bending (Backman and Goldsmith, 1978). In a perforating impact, the theoretical possibilities are much more complex. As Backman and Goldsmith (1978) have eloquently argued, these result from a number of mechanisms, all of which may be present but, of which, usually one predominates, complicated by factors such as material and geometric characteristics, as well as the velocity of impact. These authors listed eight such mechanisms, including stress wave fracture, radial fracture, spalling, plugging and fragmentation (Fig. 3.14a–e) associated with bullet deformation. Perforation without fragmentation or deformation may be associated with petaling (outfolding), infolding or ductile wound deformation (Fig. 3.14f–h).

The fact that ballistic impact is such an extremely transient event makes it difficult to apply the fundamental laws of mechanics to its interpretation. Phenomenologically, bony injury can be described as follows: because bone is denser and less elastic than its surrounding tissues, both direct impact and cavitation pressure can cause bony fracture. In the case of direct impact, a threshold velocity of around 200 ft/s (61 m/s) is thought to be required to effect penetration (Sellier and Kneubuehl, 1994). Entry wounds produced by undeformed projectiles that impact bone at right angles are usually round (described as *drill holes* by Huelke and Darling, 1964), whereas exit wounds tend to be larger and funnel shaped.

In round bones, the entrance wound is typically associated with butterfly-shaped radiating fractures (Fig. 3.15), which are usually absent in flat bone wounds (Fig. 3.16). It is thought that, because a long bone is in fact a hollow organ surrounded by hard and brittle walls, ballistic injury will be caused by cavity formation in the marrow, with splintering of tissue and a resultant permanent bony defect as remnant of the shot channel. In contrast, in a flat bone, the presence of a cancellous core serves to dissipate energy, thus preventing fracture of the bone. For a given type of bullet fired at the same distance, the resultant tissue damage will depend heavily on two factors: firstly, the location of the point of impact and, secondly, the elasticity of the tissues

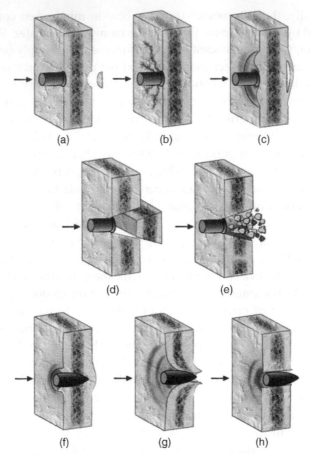

Figure 3.14 Theoretical penetration mechanisms associated with bullet deformation: (a) initial compressive wave fracture; (b) radial fracture; (c) spalling; (d) plugging; (e) fragmentation. Non-deformation may theoretically be associated with: (f) petaling or outfolding; (g) infolding; (h) ductile wound deformation. (Adapted from Backman and Goldsmith, 1978; Goldsmith, 2001.)

involved. The more flexible the tissue is, the less damage will result, simply because more energy will be transferred to the stretch mechanism (for more detail, see Sellier and Kneubuehl, 1994; Fackler, 1996; Karger, 2008).

The difficulties encountered in formulating a satisfactory biomechanical explanation of bony wounding are compounded by the fact that bones, and projectiles potentially shot into them, are so highly variable and non-homogeneous and that massive stresses are generated within an infinitesimal time span. Several studies have investigated this issue, but many questions remain. For instance, to what extent is bony damage due to compression and wedging of the impacting bullet? What is the role of thermal energy in bony wounding? What happens when the projectile deforms or fragments (as it is often designed to do)?

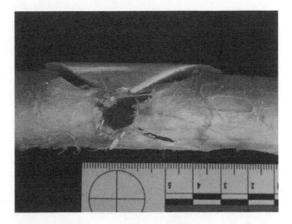

Figure 3.15 Butterfly-shaped fractures radiating from a bullet entrance wound in fresh deer bone. (Image: D. Kieser)

In answer to the first question, Shattock (1923) argued that the impacting force of the bullet transmits intense compressive force in front of the rapidly advancing projectile, which is associated with wedging and lateral compression of the bone. As we have seen, this results in a sharp, circular wound on the outer bony table, with either radiating fractures in round bones, or a conoidal exit defect in flat bones. The latter may be described as follows: a collar of melted debris on the surface of the bone (Zone I), followed by a sharply defined wound track (Zone II) and a funnel-shaped, externally bevelled exit wound, referred to as the spall (Zone III) (Fig. 3.17). How are these zones related to the biomechanical principles that surround impact? Woodward (1987) offered an early explanation in terms of two fundamental principles: the law of deformation propagation within the target material, and the law of energy conservation. They suggested that, at impact, a plug of target tissue is formed ahead of the projectile. Together, the indenter and its plug shear the surrounding tissue into a cylindrical shape. This of course begs the question: how is the conical exit wound generated?

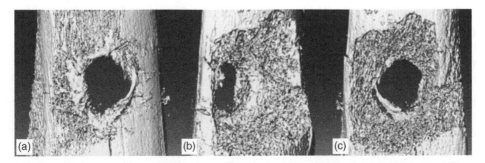

Figure 3.16 Three-dimensional CT-scan images of an experimental bullet hole through a pig rib: (a) entrance wound; (b) 45°; (c) exit wound. Note a collar of wound debris around the entrance wound, and the flared exit wound.

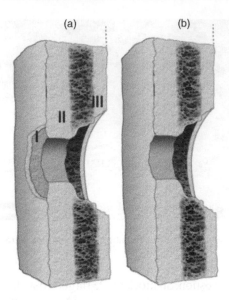

Figure 3.17 Characteristic morphology of a gunshot wound to flat bone. Zone I consists of a collar of melted debris at the entrance. Zone II is a sharply defined shot channel, followed by Zone III, a funnel-shaped exit hole. Image (a) is the appearance in a fresh bone, (b) in a weathered bone (the collar of debris is lost).

In a recent morphoscopic study, Kieser *et al.* (2011) found evidence for two processes: heat and brittle fracture. Because bone is a brittle, rigid system, there is no response time at the time of impact. The projectile punches a hole and in the process generates heat that deforms and smoothes the contact surface in Zone II (the heat zone). Soon, however, the bone starts fracturing in a brittle fashion, ripping out the cone-shaped exit cavity (Zone III, rip-out zone). Interestingly, no evidence was found for bony compression along the shot path. These authors hypothesised that the impacting projectile initiates tensile stress trajectories that radiate into the substance of the bone. This, together with deformation of the bullet, results in compressional waves spreading out in front of the bullet and its plug of bone. Progressive penetration, together with the accumulation of material in front of the deforming bullet and stress waves that radiate from it, results in the characteristic brittle fracture seen in the bevelled exit wound. Of course, not all impacts result in internal bevelling. The main limitation of bullet impact studies is that they cannot fully account for the problems of pitch and yaw of the projectile. Using non-deformable steel spheres with differing impact velocities, Huelke *et al.* (1967) showed that low-energy impacts resulted in drill-hole fractures of the distal femur, whereas high-energy impacts resulted in enlargement of the projectile path and also the exit hole.

The question now arises: what if the bullet passes in close proximity to the bone? Can it still fracture the bone? The answer is yes, and there are two reasons for this: firstly, there is a shock wave generated by the projectile as it travels through the soft tissue that surrounds the bone, and, secondly, there are powerful forces of inertia that are generated by a laterally spreading temporary cavity (Sellier and Kneubuehl, 1994).

Here we must briefly pause and discuss the concept of temporary cavity formation, first described by Woodruff in 1898. As a bullet penetrates the body, it rips its way through the soft tissue. This channel, made up of tissue destroyed by direct contact with the bullet, is called the *permanent cavity* (Fig. 3.18). Its diameter depends on the calibre of the bullet as well as its fragmentation or deformation. In addition to crushing the tissue, the projectile also sends out pressure waves perpendicular to its line of flight. These result in a forceful and rapid increase in lateral pressure that will violently stretch the neighbouring tissue. This compression of tissue creates a *temporary cavity* (Fig. 3.18). While the outward stretch of tissue around the permanent cavity will result in tearing and laceration, the viscoelastic strength of this tissue also dissipates energy, eventually resulting in a collapse of the temporary cavity. For a given tissue, the volume of the temporary cavity is proportional to the energy transferred by the missile, and can reach a maximum size up to 40 times the diameter of the bullet (Amato *et al.*, 1974). Once the bullet has passed through the tissue, the temporary cavity vibrates with diminishing amplitude until all that remains is the original permanent cavity associated with the wound tract. Thus, as a rule, low-velocity projectiles generate small temporary cavitations, and bullets travelling at high velocity generate larger cavities. High-velocity projectiles also generate compressive shock waves that progress ahead of the bullet. Both processes, probably acting sequentially, can cause bony fracture, although this is considered to be a rare event (Fackler, 1996).

Bullet velocity also plays a role in the morphological appearance of contact wounds to the cranium. Here it is important to remember that the skull is a hard, bony covering of what is essentially a jelly-like interior. The brain and its fluids (cerebrospinal and blood), being mostly water, are incompressible. Hence, a contact gunshot to the head from a high-velocity projectile will result in major cranial fracturing together with outward displacement of large portions of the skull (Waters, 2008). In contrast, low-velocity contact wounds are characterised by fracturing without blowout.

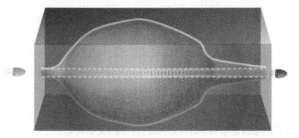

Figure 3.18 Schematic diagram of the permanent cavity along the path of a bullet (stippled lines) and its associated temporary cavity (solid lines). The permanent cavity is the actual bullet track through the tissue, while the temporary cavity is due to lateral stretching of surrounding tissues.

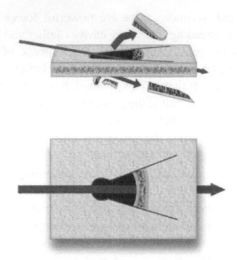

Figure 3.19 Supposed biomechanical explanation for the generation of a keyhole defect after a tangential shot to the head (after Dixon, 1982).

Bony penetration by a projectile may be considered from four points of view: firstly, the velocity of the impact; secondly, material characteristics of the bony target; thirdly, the material characteristics of the bullet; and, finally, the angle of the impact. So far we have dealt with the first two categories. The material configuration of projectiles is a hugely important, complex and ever-changing subject about which numerous texts have been written, and falls outside the scope of this book. Angle of impact and its relationship to bony wound morphology is controversial and a much disputed subject. Classically, entrance wounds from perpendicular gunshots are round or ovoid in shape, with sharply defined outer margins and internal bevelling (Fig. 3.17). While some have accepted the shape of this bevelling to be an indicator of the direction of fire, others have not (for discussion, see Quatrehomme and Iscan, 1998). One example of where entrance wound morphology may be useful is in the diagnosis of tangential shots to the head. Here the projectile is thought to punch out an ovoid entrance defect, simultaneously creating a roughly trapezoid hole with external bevelling at its base along the line of fire (Fig. 3.19), resulting in what is described as a keyhole defect (Dixon, 1982). However, size and shape of cranial gunshot wounds are notoriously difficult to interpret biomechanically, as is illustrated in Figure 3.20, showing a keyhole defect with an in-fractured, rather than an out-fractured, trapezoid segment.

3.7 Living versus postmortem fracture

Distinguishing living (antemortem) fractures from those that occurred at the time of death (perimortem), or more importantly after-death (postmortem) damage, is

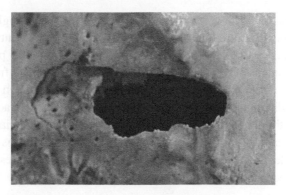

Figure 3.20 Keyhole defect in the skull of a 36-year-old male. Note the in-fracture of the trapezoid segment.

obviously important in forensics because it facilitates reconstruction of circumstances surrounding the death of a victim, particularly where full skeletonisation is involved. As we have seen, bone consists of a mineral phase (hydroxyapatite) and an organic matrix (mainly Type I collagen). While mineral contributes to bone strength and stiffness, and collagen to its toughness (Wang *et al.*, 2002), there are other factors to consider when thinking of bony fracture. These include its gross anatomy (macrostructural features such as its shape and size), microstructure (microarchitectural features such as trabecular design) and the presence of microfractures. There is, however, another important factor: bone is a fluid-imbibed material and, hence, its water content is critical to its mechanical behaviour. Nyman *et al.* (2006) examined the mechanical effects of dehydration on human cadaveric bone. They noted that intrabony water was not only found within the vascular canals and canaliculi (Fig. 3.1), but also within the collagen matrix itself. In other words, water distributed within bone consists not only of mobile water, but also structurally bound water. Clearly, mobile water requires less energy to evaporate than the removal of water trapped inside the collagen matrix. Interestingly, water loss caused by drying at room temperature actually increased bone strength, possibly because the stiffness of collagen increases (Pineri *et al.*, 1978). However, there was a degree of loss of plasticity. When sufficient energy was applied in the form of high temperature dehydration, bone strength markedly decreased. The decrease in work to fracture means that water bound in the mineral phase affects the toughness of bone and, hence, also the energy-absorbing capacity of bone.

Forensic biologists have long assumed that wet (perimortem) fractures may be distinguished from dry (postmortem) bony trauma by features such as the fracture edge or fracture angle. Whereas fracture edges of wet bones tend to be sharp, smooth and often bevelled, dry fractures are said to be jagged-edged and at right angles to the long axis of the bone (for review, see Moraitis and Spiliopoulou, 2006). Intriguingly, a study by Wheatley (2008) in deer femora suggests that these characteristics may in fact be unreliable in differentiating postmortem from perimortem fracture. Whereas transverse fractures and right-angled edges were unique to dry bone fractures, they were only rarely observed. Butterfly fractures, thought to be diagnostic of wet fractures, were reported in both postmortem and perimortem specimens. The author did find, however, that helical fracture patterns, in other words a radial fracture circling the shaft, were only seen in wet bones.

The ability to distinguish between peri- and postmortem bony fracture allows one to determine the timing of the injury. Moreover, the ability to associate a bony injury to the time of death is one of the most significant considerations in the forensic evaluation of a fatality (Sauer, 1998). Unfortunately, with the research currently available such reconstructions remain speculative at best.

3.8 Bone fracture in infants

The report by Currey (2003) of his investigation into the mechanical properties of femora at different ages showed an important distinction between the modulus of elasticity and impact strength. Importantly, he found that during the early years of life the modulus of elasticity increased markedly. Bending strength also increased, but less dramatically. Impact strength, however, decreased sharply. These changes he attributed directly to the degree of mineralisation of the bone: immature bone was progressing towards full mineralisation and, hence, was stronger in impact than adult bone. Children's bones are not stiff, but are unusually impact resistant. Moreover, while adult bone is stronger in compression than in tension, the opposite is true in children: immature bone is weaker in compression, thus resulting in different fracture morphologies compared to adults (Ogden, 2000). In spite of the foregoing, we still have only a limited knowledge of the biomechanics of immature bones. Yet children of one year or younger are at the greatest risk of non-accidental injury, with an estimated 40–80% of long bone fractures attributable to child abuse (but see Schwend *et al.*, 2000). Clearly the fracture *per se* is not diagnostic of abuse; it is merely a reflection of the action of the stress generated on the bone, as well as its ability to resist such stress. Understanding the biomechanics of bony injuries in children does, however, allow one to evaluate the stated injury history in terms of the magnitude and direction of force, as well as the expected response from the bone (Pierce *et al.*, 2004).

We know that the strength of bone is related to its mineral density. Because children's bones have a lower mineral content, they are elastic and hence, can absorb relatively more energy before permanent damage, in the form of fracture, ensues. There are a number of commonly recognised fracture types in immature bones.

Spiral fractures occur when torque is applied to a long bone (Fig. 3.21). Debate continues about the relationship of spiral fracturing and non-accidental injury in children. These fractures are known to occur with tripping or falling and are thus not diagnostic of abuse (Frazier, 2003).

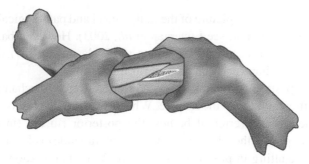

Figure 3.21 Spiral fracture of a baby's arm subjected to torque. (Adapted from Bilo *et al.*, 2010.)

Buckle fractures in children differ from those in adults. Because immature bone tends to fail in compression before tension, these fractures result typically from axial loading and are usually found at the metaphyseal ends of long bones where buckling is circumferential. When they do occur in the midshaft region (diaphyseal), they are usually associated with bending, and a unicortical buckling results (Fig. 3.13).

Transverse fractures usually result from direct, high-energy impacts to a long bone, resulting in a fracture line perpendicular to the long axis of the bone (Fig. 3.13). Lower energy impacts may result in incomplete, or *greenstick* injuries. The literature suggests that transverse fractures are more common in abusive trauma (Scherl *et al.*, 2000).

Classic metaphysical lesions (*CMLs*) are thought to be associated with yanking a child up by the arms, and may be highly associative with abuse (Pierce *et al.*, 2004). Because immature spongy bone does not contain Haversian systems, shearing stresses at the metaphyseal angle can result in a planar fracture of this region. This type of fracture is also often associated with violent shaking by an extremity.

Rib fractures in older children are mostly the result of falls or motor vehicle impact injuries, but these are highly unusual injuries in infants and are strongly correlated with abuse. It has been suggested that a tight hold around the infant's chest, together with chest encirclement and compression, may result in fractures to the anterior, lateral and posterior aspects of the ribs (Fig. 3.22). Numerous clinical surveys and case

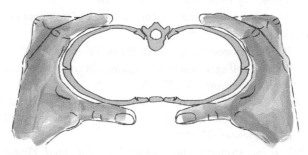

Figure 3.22 Antero-posterior compression of the ribs in an infant.

reports have given us a clear picture of the radiological and pathological appearances of such fractures (for review, see Lonergan *et al.*, 2003). However, barring a single experimental study on three rabbits (Kleinman and Schlesinger, 1997), there has been no systematic biomechanical evaluation of rib fractures.

During antero-posterior compression of the chest, different mechanical forces are generated on different parts of the ribcage. What is hypothesised is that, because the ribs are attached to the vertebral bodies, the posterior rib arc (in other words, the paravertebral part of the rib, proximal to the rib tubercle) is levered against the vertebral body, resulting in posterior rib fracture. What is not known, however, is the force required for such fracture. We also do not know what the differences in fracture mechanisms are between slow (squeezing) or fast (high-energy impact) forces applied to the ribs. Indeed, we do not even know how infantile ribs behave under different loading regimes.

References

Amato JJ, Billy LJ, Lawson NS, Rich NM. 1974. High velocity missile energy: an experimental study of the retentive forces of tissue. *American Journal of Surgery* **127**:454–9.

Backman ME, Goldsmith W. 1978. The mechanics of penetration of projectiles into targets. *International Journal of Engineering Science* **16**:1–99.

Bartlett C. 2003. Clinical update: gunshot wound ballistics. *Clinical Orthopaedics and Related Research* **408**:28–57.

Bilo RAC, Robben SGF, van Rijn RR. 2010. *Forensic Aspects of Paediatric Fractures*. Springer, Heidelberg.

Burgess WH, Maciag T. 1989. The heparin binding (fibroblast) growth factor family of proteins. *Annual Reviews of Biochemistry* **58**:575–606.

Cullinane DM, Einhorn TA. 2002. Biomechanics of bone. In: *Principles of Bone Biology*, 2nd Edition. Bilezikian JP, Raisz LG, Rodan GA (Editors). Academic Press, San Diego: pp. 17–32.

Currey JD. 1969. Physical characteristics affecting the tensile failure properties of compact bone. *Journal of Biomechanics* **23**:837–44.

Currey JD. 1999. What determines the bending strength of compact bone? *Journal of Experimental Biology* **202**:2495–503.

Currey JD. 2002. *Bones*. Princeton University Press, Princeton.

Currey JD. 2003. Role of collagen and other organics in the mechanical properties of bone. *Osteoporosis International* **14**:29–36.

DiMaio VJM. 1998. *Gunshot Wounds*, 2nd Edition. CRC Press, Boca Raton, FL.

Dixon DS. 1982. Keyhole lesions in gunshot wounds of the skull and direction of fire. *Journal of Forensic Sciences* **27**:555–6.

Einhorn TA. 1992. Bone strength: the bottom line. *Calcified Tissue International* **51**:333–9.

Fackler ML. 1996. Gunshot wound review. *Annals of Emergency Medicine* **28**:194–203.

Filer JM. 1992. Head injuries in Egypt and Nubia: a comparison of skulls from Giza and Kerma. *Journal of Egyptian Archaeology* **78**:281–5.

Fratzl P. 2008. When the cracks begin to show. *Nature Materials* **7**:610–12.

Frazier LD. 2003. Child abuse or mimic? *Consultant Paediatricians* **2**:212–15.

Goldsmith W. 2001. *Impact*. Dover Publications, New York.

Huelke DF, Darling JH. 1964. Bone fractures produced by bullets. *Journal of Forensic Sciences* **9**:461–9.

Huelke DF, Buege LJ, Harger JH. 1967. Bone fractures produced by high velocity impacts. *American Journal of Anatomy* **120**:123–32.

Kanz F, Grossschmidt K. 2006. Head injuries in Roman gladiators. *Forensic Science International* **160**:207–16.

Karger B. 2008. Forensic ballistics. *Forensic Pathology Reviews* **5**:139–72.

Kieser JA, Tahere J, Agnew C, Kieser DC, Duncan W, Swain MV, Reeves MT. 2011. Morphoscopic analysis of experimentally produced bony wounds from low-velocity ballistic impact. *Forensic Science, Medicine, and Pathology* **7**:322–32.

Kleinman PK, Schlesinger AE. 1997. Mechanical factors associated with posterior rib fractures: laboratory and case studies. *Pediatric Radiology* **27**:87–91.

Koester KJ, Ager JW, Ritchie RO. 2008. The true toughness of human cortical bone measured with realistically short cracks. *Nature Materials* **7**:672–7.

Launey ME, Buehler MJ, Ritchie RO. 2010. On the mechanistic origins of toughness in bone. *Annual Reviews of Material Research* **40**:25–53.

Lonergan GL, Baker AM, Morey MK, Boos SC. 2003. Child abuse: radiologic-pathologic correlation. *Radiographics* **23**:811–45.

Lovell NC. 1997. Trauma analysis in paleopathology. *Yearbook of Physical Anthropology* **40**:139–70.

Meikle MC. 2002. *Craniofacial Development, Growth and Evolution*. Bateson Publishing, Bressingham, Norfolk.

Ming L, Yu-Yuan M, Ring-Xiang F, Tian-Shun F. 1988. The characteristics of pressure waves generated in the soft tissue by impact and its contribution to indirect bone fracture. *Journal of Trauma* **28**:S104–9.

Moraitis K, Spiliopoulou C. 2006. Identification and differential diagnosis of peri-mortem blunt force trauma in tubular long bones. *Forensic Science, Medicine, and Pathology* **2**:221–9.

Nagaraja S, Couse TL, Guldberg RE. 2005. Trabecular bone microdamage and microstructural stresses under uniaxial compression. *Journal of Biomechanics* **38**:707–16.

Nalla RK, Kinney JH, Ritchie RO. 2003. Mechanistic fracture criteria for the failure of human cortical bone. *Nature Materials* **2**:164–8.

Nyman JS, Roy A, Shen X, Acuna RL, Tyler JH, Wang X. 2006. The influence of water removal on the strength and toughness of cortical bone. *Journal of Biomechanics* **39**:931–8.

Ogden JA. 2000. *Skeletal Injury in the Child*. Springer, New York.

Peterlink H, Roschger P, Klaushofer K, Fratzl P. 2006. From brittle to ductile fracture in bone. *Nature Materials* **5**:52–5.

Pierce MC, Bertocci GE, Vogeley E, Moreland MS. 2004. Evaluating long bone fractures in children: a biomechanical approach with illustrative cases. *Child Abuse and Neglect* **28**:505–24.

Pineri MH, Escoubes M, Roche G. 1978. Water-collagen interactions: calorimetric and mechanical experiments. *Biopolymers* **17**:2799–815.

Quatrehomme G, Iscan MY. 1998. Analysis of beveling in gunshot entrance wounds. *Forensic Science International* **93**:45–60.

Rho JY, Kuhn-Spearing L, Zioupos P. 1998. Mechanical properties and the hierarchical structure of bone. *Medical Engineering and Physics* **20**:92–102.

Ritchie RO. 1999. Mechanisms of fatigue-crack propagation in ductile or brittle solids. *International Journal of Fracture* **100**:55–83.

Ritchie RO. 2010. How does human bone resist fracture? *Annals of the New York Academy of Sciences* **1192**:72–80.

Sauer NJ. 1998. The timing of injuries and manner of death: distinguishing among antemortem, perimortem and postmortem trauma. In: *Forensic Osteology*. Reichs KJ (Editor), Charles Thomas, Springfield, IL: pp. 321–32.

Scherl SA, Miller L, Lively N, Russinoff S, Sullivan CM, Tornetta P. 2000. Accidental and non-accidental femur fractures in children. *Clinical Orthopaedics and Related Research* **376**:96–105.

Schwend RM, Worth C, Johnston A. 2000. Femur shaft fractures in toddlers and young children: rarely from child abuse. *Journal of Paediatric Orthopaedics* **20**:475–81.

Sellier KG, Kneubuehl BP. 1994. *Wound Ballistics and the Scientific Background*. Elsevier, Amsterdam.

Shattock SG. 1923. The disruptive phenomena in gunshot injuries: their physics. *Proceedings of the Royal Society of Medicine* **16**:17–34.

Sugita H, Oka M, Toguchida J, Nakamura T, Ueo T, Hayami T. 1999. Anisotropy of osteoporotic cancellous bone. *Bone* **24**:513–16.

Turner CH. 2006. Bone strength: current concepts. *Annals of the New York Academy of Sciences* **1068**:429–46.

Turner CH, Burr DB. 1993. Basic biomechanical measurements of bone: a tutorial. *Bone* **14**:595–608.

Wang X, Shen X, Li X, Agraval CM. 2002. Age related changes in the collagen network and toughness of bone. *Bone* **31**:1–7.

Waters CJ. 2008. Gunfire injuries. In: *Skeletal Trauma*. Kimmerle EH, Baraybar JP (Editors). CRC Press, Boca Raton: pp. 385–400.

Weibull W. 1951. A statistical distribution function of wide applicability. *Journal of Applied Mechanics* **18**:293–305.

Wheatley BP. 2008. Perimortem or postmortem bone fractures? *An experimental study of fracture patterns in deer femora. Journal of Forensic Sciences* **53**:69–72.

Woodruff CE. 1898. The causes of the explosive effect of modern small caliber bullets. *New York Medical Journal* **67**:593–601.

Woodward RL. 1987. A structural model for thin plate perforation by normal impact of blunt projectiles. *International Journal of Impact Engineering* **6**:129–40.

4

Biomechanics of skin and soft tissue trauma

Jules Kieser

4.1 Structure of skin

Skin is the largest organ in the body and consists of three main layers, referred to as the epidermis, dermis and hypodermis (Fig. 4.1). The deepest layer of the skin is the subcutaneous layer of fat, called the *hypodermis*. Its thickness varies considerably within individuals, depending on site (sadly more fat on the abdomen), and between individuals (sex and ancestry play a part). Subcutaneous fat consists of white adipose tissue (about 75%), water (20%) and protein (5%). The white adipose tissue consists of lipid-filled adipocytes that are held in a framework of collagen.

The *dermis* overlays the hypodermis and is a dense fibroelastic connective tissue layer of about 1–3 mm in thickness (Montagna and Parakkal, 1974), thus forming the bulk of normal skin. This layer is in turn divided into a deeper reticular dermis and a more superficial papillary dermis, which contains both elastic and collagen fibres, as well as hair follicles, sebaceous and sweat glands. The dermal layer provides structural strength to the skin and acts as a water storage organ (60–70% by volume consists of water). Within the dermis, collagen is the dominant fibrous component (30% by volume) and gives skin its material integrity at high load levels (Sanders *et al.*, 1995). Collagen molecules (Type I) within a fibre are staggered to allow a quarter-length overlap between adjacent molecules. Cross-links between fibrils are critical in force dissipation. Together with reticulin fibres (collagen Type III) and proteoglycans, collagen plays a vital role in determining the biomechanical properties of skin, and hence its ability to absorb external forces. Delicately interwoven reticulin fibres form a loose network for tissue fluids to pass through; a configuration that is essential for the exchange of nutrients and metabolites.

In contrast to collagen and reticulin, elastin fibres are thin, forming a meshlike network within the skin. Elastin maintains mechanical integrity at low loads, enabling skin to recoil at low force levels – an ability that is progressively lost with advancing age.

The superficial *epidermis* is a highly organised structure consisting of outwardly migrating cells, called keratinocytes, which are formed by constant division of cells at the deepest level, the stratum basale. The epidermis is an avascular layer of varying thickness (think of underarm compared with sole of foot) and acts as a protective layer against physical, thermal, chemical and radiation injury. It is also the first line of defence against microbial attack. To do this, it has a high cellular

Forensic Biomechanics, First Edition. Jules Kieser, Michael Taylor and Debra Carr.
© 2013 John Wiley & Sons, Ltd. Published 2013 by John Wiley & Sons, Ltd.

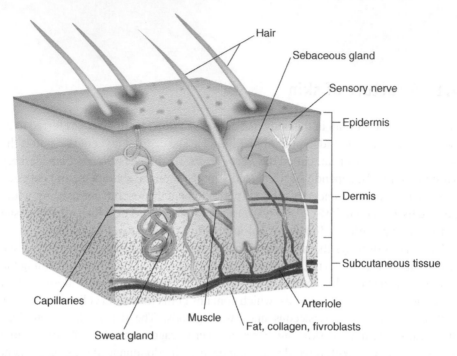

Hair

Sebaceous gland

Sensory nerve

Epidermis

Dermis

Subcutaneous tissue

Capillaries

Arteriole

Muscle

Fat, collagen, fivroblasts

Sweat gland

Figure 4.1   Normal skin in cross-section, showing the three principal layers.

turnover attained by cells constantly migrating from their origin in the stratum basale, toward the skin surface. During migration, these cells do two things: firstly, they accumulate a tough fibrous protein called keratin; and secondly, they die. This results in a superficial layer of tough, dead cells arranged like tiles, and referred to as the *stratum corneum* (Fig. 4.2). These cells become progressively flattened, before they are lost. The entire process takes about a month.

The interface between the superficial epidermis and its underlying dermis consists of a wavy basement membrane, with tiny, finger-like projections (rete ridges) that anchor the two layers together (Briggaman, 1982). This acts as a permeable barrier between the vascular dermis and the avascular epidermis, and provides adherence between the two tissues. Skin has a rich blood supply which

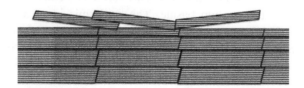

Figure 4.2   Diagram of the tiled arrangement of cells of the stratum corneum. Dead cells, packed with tough keratin fibres, become progressively flattened toward the surface, where they slough off.

contributes greatly to its healing ability, but at the same time also allows the skin to bleed profusely when cut. It should be remembered, however, that the density of blood vessels in the papillary dermis varies according to location, age and function (Pasyk *et al.*, 1989). These are particularly dense in the skin of the scalp and fingertips, and less dense in the palm and sole.

4.2   Mechanical properties of skin

Skin varies enormously with position, age and ethnicity; hence, when thinking of skin in relation to trauma, one should adopt a wide approach by considering how a particular insult is transmitted to underlying tissues. Broadly speaking, three tissues are involved: skin, adipose (fat) tissue and muscle. Because of widely differing biomechanical properties in respect to water content, anisotropy and viscoelasticity, it is extremely hard to determine how these tissues will behave when a traumatic force is applied to the skin. For instance, Le *et al.* (1984) measured pressures at different layers of soft tissue over a pig hind-leg and found that the internal pressure on the trochanteric eminence was several times greater than the surface pressure. However, Dodd and Gross (1991) measured interstitial pressure in pigs when pressure was applied to the skin over the wing of the ilium, and showed that only about one-third of the pressure was dissipated as soft tissue moved away from the load.

Skin is a three-dimensional matrix of loosely arranged collagen and elastin fibres in an amorphous gel of ground substance. Whereas collagen accounts for its tensile strength and stiffness, elastin is responsible for the recoil after deformation. Skin is mobile, because when it is relaxed, the collagen fibres form a convoluted and randomly dispersed network, separated by tissue fluid and ground substance (Gibson *et al.*, 1965). At low stress levels, skin acts like an elastic material, but, as stress increases, it becomes increasingly viscoelastic with the stress/strain relationship becoming time dependent. In other words, when subject to deformation, skin generates a low resistant force which is time independent (i.e. elastic and independent of the loading history) and a higher resistive force that is time dependent (i.e. viscous and dependent on the strain rate). When it is stretched, collagen fibres straighten out and align along the applied force. At maximum stretch, most of the ground substance and tissue fluid is displaced, giving skin its characteristic tri-phasic stress/strain curve (Fig. 4.3). Initially, the collagen network offers little resistance, with elastic fibres dominating the response to an applied load. This low-stiffness region is followed by a dramatic increase in stiffness as collagen fibres begin to resist deformation. A linear phase ensues, dominated by the behaviour of the collagen network, during which collagen fibres aligned parallel to the force direction provide increasing stiffness by stretch resistance. This high-stiffness phase is followed by a yield region associated with fibrillar slippage, before failure occurs (Payne, 1991; Silver *et al.*, 2001a).

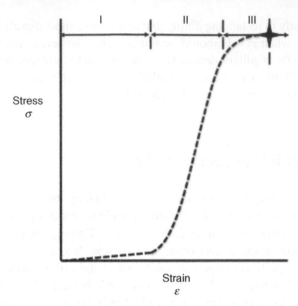

Figure 4.3 Typical tri-phasic, J-shaped stress/strain curve for skin: Phase I (low stiffness, toe region) represents stretching of elastic fibres with the collagen network offering little resistance; in Phase II (linear response), collagen fibres begin to resist deformation; followed by Phase III, a yield region, dominated by defibrillation and eventual failure.

What this means, in essence, is that a force applied to the skin is in part dissipated by the stretching of elastic fibres followed by viscous sliding of collagen fibres as they are reoriented along the direction of the force, which accounts for the large extensibility of the skin. Reticular fibres, together with returning fluid, ensure rapid shape recovery once the force is removed (Dunn and Silver, 1983). Being visco-elastic, the nature of deformation, and of course recovery, will depend on the rate of loading as well as on its magnitude. Whereas rapid, short loads result in elastic deformation associated with minimum creep and rapid recovery, prolonged loading leads to conspicuous creep with delayed recovery.

Given its primary biological function, an understanding of how skin behaves under traumatic loads must begin with an understanding of the perspective of stress and strain. Figure 4.3 shows a classical J-shaped stress/strain curve, characteristic of a tough material such as skin (Gordon, 2003). The fact that an initial, small increase in load will result in a large extension can be verified by tugging down on one's earlobe. While it is easy to stretch initially, it becomes rapidly more difficult. Note, also, that loading and unloading is reversible. In other words, under normal conditions of use, energy used in deformation is returned when the load is removed. During the low-modulus, toe region (Phase I), elastic fibres stretch and wavy collagen fibres straighten (Oxlund *et al.*, 1988). This is followed by a linear region characterised by stretching and slippage of collagen molecules situated within cross-linked collagen fibres (Silver *et al.*, 2001b). Phase III is the viscous yield and failure region, dominated by slippage and defibrillation of the collagen. The question now emerges: how is energy stored or lost in skin under impact? Phases I and II reflect energy stored when elastic and collagen fibres stretch, and Phase III the energy lost through slippage. On stretching, skin behaves almost in a tendon-like fashion, with the slope of the stress/strain curve independent of strain rate. In contrast, at the viscous Phase III, skin becomes thixotropic (skin behaves like a solid at normal stress, but when squeezed, it shear-thins).

J-shaped stress curves have become somewhat of a catch-all notion of extreme toughness because of the following reasons: firstly, the toe region (Phase I) is characterised by large extension for low stress, incompatible with fracture initiation; secondly, the linear zone (II) means that increased stiffness requires large stresses, hence larger loads are required for fracture; finally, the area under the concave curve is clearly smaller than that under an r-shaped curve (e.g. of bone), hence there is less energy available for crack propagation. Remember, though, that this toughness does not apply to situations where fracture energy is geometry dependent. A classic example is in the so-called trouser-tear test, which does not depend on the elastic properties of the material tested (Kendall and Fuller, 1987). Skin and other biological materials do not appear to be extremely tough in this test.

Although human skin is compliant, it is also tough and resilient. Its bio-mechanical properties vary between and within individuals. They also vary with direction. This is because skin is normally pre-stressed; in other words, it is subjected to continuous internal tension. This stress is anisotropic, because it is necessary to accommodate stretching required during movements of the body. More than a century ago Karl Langer documented these directional variations in the properties of skin by punching circular holes in cadaver skin. He observed that the holes became elliptical. By drawing lines through all the long axes of each of the ellipses, he noticed a definite patterning of cleavage lines (Langer, 1861; Gibson, 1978; Langer, 1978a,b,c). Local differences in pre-stress directionality result from bundles of fibrous tissue in the reticular dermis and, in general, tend to be horizontal in the neck and trunk, and longitudinal in the limbs (Cox, 1941). Stab wound morphology typically varies according to its position relative to these stress lines, which have become known as Langer's lines (Byard *et al.*, 2005). Importantly, however, Langer's lines are not a static feature, but are dynamic, which means that movement may affect the appearance of incisive wounds (Bush *et al.*, 2007). The question now is: what is the biomechanical reason for Langer's cleavage lines? One theory is that of Ridge and Wright (1966), who postulated that Langer's lines in fact followed the direction of the general orientation of skin fibres, and that these formed a lattice parallel to Langer's lines. Hence, a cut across Langer's lines would cut more skin fibres than an incision along them and thus, would be subject to more tensile stress, resulting in a gaping wound.

4.3   Effect of age

Skin biomechanics vary regionally and also with health, body mass and age. We are all too familiar with the tight, sensitive skin of babies on the one hand and the lax, wrinkly skin of old age. Hence, recognition of these changes and their effects on the biomechanical properties of skin are important in understanding the mechanisms of wounding.

Age-related degeneration affects all areas of skin. Structural, biochemical and physiological changes associated with age all impact directly on the biomechanical properties of skin; however, data on dermal age changes are difficult to obtain because of confounders such as environmental effects or disease. With age comes epidermal thinning and flattening of the rete ridges, resulting in a weakened dermal–epidermal junction. As a consequence, older skin becomes inelastic and rigid, increasingly unable to undergo reversible deformation when subjected to even minor trauma. One of the major effects of this is the increased chance of skin trauma resulting from tangential forces (Richey *et al.*, 1988). Similarly, changes in collagen quality and arrangement result in decreased extensibility.

While numerous studies have shown that skin thickness generally decreases with age (e.g. Shuster *et al.*, 1975), some investigators have found that there is in fact an increase in facial skin thickness from about 20 to 60 years, particularly in those areas exposed to the sun (Takema *et al.*, 1994). Diridollou and co-workers (2001) studied age-related changes in human skin *in vivo* in 206 volunteers, ranging from 6 months to 90 years, and also found that skin thickness increased until maturity in both sexes. These results agreed with earlier studies that showed that, between 0 and 20 years, there was an increase in thickness, followed by a constant phase between 20 and 60 years (e.g. Escoffier *et al.*, 1980). Interestingly, they also measured Young's modulus, and compared it to what they termed the *natural stress*, which reflects the intrinsic stiffness and tension in living, pre-stressed skin. While Young's modulus increased with age, the natural pre-stress of the skin decreased; in other words, skin becomes less elastic and more viscous with age. One of the reasons for this is that the quality of the collagen changes with age. Not only do fibres appear detached, but also tend to be disrupted by areas of entanglement (Lavker *et al.*, 1986). However, these effects may, to a certain extent, be masked by excess subcutaneous fat (Boyer *et al.*, 2009).

Silver *et al.* (2002) reported significant differences in the viscosity of skin between 23-year-old and 87-year-old donors, which they attributed to a decrease in collagen fibril viscosity. However, despite numerous studies, it has not been possible to formulate an accurate picture of which changes relate to true ageing (the passage of time) or to actinic ageing (due to factors such as exposure to sunlight or smoking). An additional confounding factor is the observation that more darkly pigmented persons tend to retain younger skin properties compared to paler skinned individuals (Rawlins, 2006). This presents the forensic scientist with somewhat of a

Case 4.1   The effect of age on abrasions of the skin

Abrasions generally occur when the skin is scraped against a rough surface. The skin is both tough and elastic – biomechanical properties that are important in its function as a protective barrier to the underlying organs and tissues. With age, viscoelasticity of the skin changes, as does its ability to resist deformation. Clearly, these changes have to be borne in mind when evaluating dermal injuries.

a. The left cheek of the three-year-old girl was injured when a small dog that she had been playing with turned on her. The wounds are a combination of abrasions on the right, caused by the dog's lower incisors scraping against her skin, while the puncture marks on the left were created by the dog's upper incisors engaging the cheek as the jaws closed.

b. The left lateral aspect of the face of a 33-year-old victim of assault shows similar linearity of abrasions, in this case caused by being dragged across tar in a car park. The abrasions are clearly more superficial than those of the child, with no evidence of partial avulsion of superficial skin. Note the additional presence of a contusion beneath the left eye.

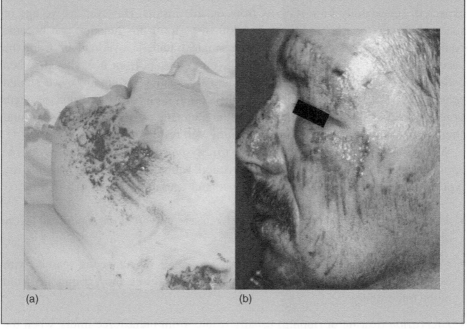

(a)   (b)

conundrum; while we anecdotally know that older skin is more fragile than younger skin, the notions of the modulus of elasticity, tone, firmness or fragility cannot be reduced to time-related change in simple physical measurements, and hence the difficulty of reconstructing traumatic events in the elderly (Kieser *et al.*, 2008a).

4.4 Wounding

One of the primary functions of skin is to protect the internal organs from mechanical trauma. This ability depends on its viscoelastic properties and its two-phase response to external forces applied to it. As stated previously, this involves a viscous component associated with energy dissipation and an elastic response associated with energy storage. When the external force exceeds these properties, skin will rupture. The level of rupture resistance of skin depends primarily on the morphology and material properties of the skin in the area of contact. Although these characteristics have been examined in a number of studies (as discussed above), no single measurement can fully describe the structural integrity of skin, nor can it reliably predict the occurrence and nature of rupture. To complicate matters, factors such as age, sex and disease can compromise skin integrity. We constantly impose dynamic mechanical stimuli on our skins during normal daily activities. Throughout our lives, our skin performs as expected, successfully protecting us from outside insults. However, as we age or succumb to disease, the ability of our skin to perform this function can become compromised. Failure can result from a single traumatic overload or from the accumulated damage of repetitive loading (think blisters from new shoes). When considering the failure of skin under traumatic loading (wounding), we should consider the forces or insults applied to the skin as well as the structural strength or resistance to failure of the skin itself. If the traumatic force exceeds the structural strength of the skin, it will fail and wounding will result.

Wounding can be defined as *damage to any part of the body caused by the application of mechanical force* (Saukko and Knight, 2004). Skin wounds are typically classified according to appearance and causation (Fig. 4.4).

- *Abrasion* (grazing or scratching) results from scraping off of the superficial layers of skin.

- *Contusion* (bruising) results from damage to small subcutaneous vessels, with extravasation of blood into the subdermal tissues. It results most commonly from blunt force injury.

- *Laceration* (tearing or ripping) usually results from blunt force injury when the full thickness of the skin is involved. It is characteristically associated with irregular wound margins, bruising and skin tagging.

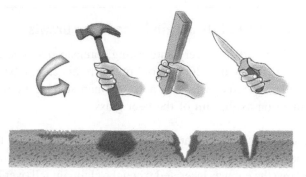

Figure 4.4 Four classical types of wounding: from left to right, *abrasion* involves scraping away of the superficial parts of the skin, *contusion* results from subcutaneous bleeding, *laceration* is typically caused by blunt force injury to the full thickness of the skin and *incisions* are cuts by sharp objects. (Adapted from Saukko and Knight, 2004.)

- *Incision* (cut) is the wound that results from cutting with a sharp object such as a knife.

- Bitemarks are complex wounds, caused by the application of teeth to the skin. Because they can involve humans and other animals, ranging in size from sharks to rodents, these are a specialised topic (see Section 4.8).

4.5 Sharp force trauma

How does an object penetrate a soft solid like skin? In 2004, Oliver Shergold and Norman Fleck of Cambridge University published the results of their experiments into this question. Their technique involved the penetration of silicone rubbers and skin by sharp-tipped and flat-bottomed cylindrical punches. Penetration experiments showed clearly that penetration mechanism depended on the geometry of the punch tip. Whereas a sharp-tipped punch wedged open a planar (Type I) crack, the blunt punch penetrated by a ring (Type II) crack, beneath which skin was deformed and a compressed plug generated. Not only was the penetration pressure of a flat-bottomed punch several times higher than that of a sharp-tipped punch of the same diameter, but perforation pressure decreased as the diameter of the sharp-tipped punch increased with increased penetration.

Stab wounds from knives or sharp instruments like screwdrivers are frequent in assault and homicide. The question that is traditionally asked when these cases go to trial is: *What was the force required to inflict this wound?* This is a difficult question that has occupied the minds of a number of forensic scientists since the first publication of Knight's study in 1975. In this study, he used an instrumented knife attached to a spring balance to create penetrating wounds near the lines of autopsy incisions in cadavers. Importantly, he concluded the following.

Case 4.2   Cutting and thrusting in barroom brawls

Barroom brawls can deliver very interesting forensic outcomes. Image (a) shows a patterned injury in a 26-year-old male. In this case, a beer glass was forcibly applied to his left eye, leaving a well-demarcated laceration of roughly the same dimension as the rim of the beer glass.

The case shown in (b) is less clear-cut. In this case, a 44-year-old man alleged that his earlobe had been bitten off during a fight. The supposed assailant, in turn, claimed that the ear was lacerated when the claimant fell over his own feet and his head came into forceful contact with a metal bar stool. In this case the analysis of the alleged bite was complicated by the complexity of the earlobe, in the sense that it consisted of a sandwich of skin and cartilage, each with its own biomechanical characteristics.

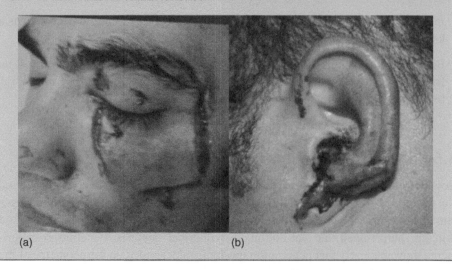

(a)   (b)

- The most important determinant of penetration was the sharpness of the blade tip. A highly whetted tip needed but the pressure of a finger to penetrate skin.

- The greater the speed of impact, the less force is required for penetration.

- The skin is a reservoir of resistance. Once it penetrates the skin, no further force is required for penetration, unless a bone or calcified tissue is encountered.

These results were confirmed by Green (1978), who used a spring-based instrumented knife to determine forces required to produce wounds. However, neither author was able to directly measure these forces, because their apparatus did not incorporate force transducers housed inside the knives. Subsequent studies by Jones *et al.* (1994) and O'Callaghan *et al.* (1999) have questioned the last of Knight's three

Case 4.3   Offensive and defensive wounds in a dog attack

This case illustrates the defensive wounds sustained on the arm of a female victim of a dog attack. The round punch-marks on the forearm show where the victim tried to fend off the large dog as it tried to grab hold of her (a). The subsequent fatal injuries to the front of the neck resulted from offensive wounds, when the dog typically surged and attacked her face and throat (b, c).

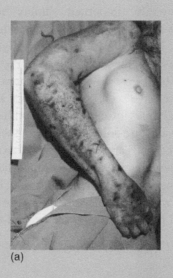

(a)

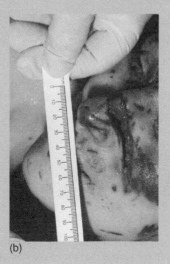

(b)

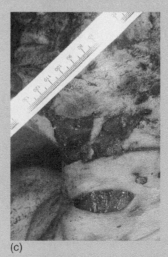

(c)

principal findings; they found secondary pressure peaks corresponding to the penetration of underlying tissue. In answer to the leading question – what force is required – they found that skin requires between 35 N and 55 N to penetrate, with fat and muscle requiring 35–40 N, and fat 1–2 N. Chadwick and colleagues (1999) investigated knife stab attacks using a six-camera motion analysis system to measure velocity and derive energy and momentum during the approach phase of an assault. They used three styles of thrust: a short upwards lunge, a horizontal sweep and an overhand stab. The highest cutting forces were reported for the overhand stab at approximately 300 N. These results, however, need to be seen in the light of their volunteer participants. All were large, muscular police officers trained in self-defence.

Screwdriver wounds are also important, simply because this is an easily concealed, multiple use weapon. Two recent studies have investigated the bio-mechanics of such attacks. Kieser *et al.* (2008b) investigated wounding patterns of five common screwdrivers (straight, star, Robertson, Pozidriv and Phillips) using a drop tube and pig heads. There were obvious differences between the straight head and the other types. As we have seen, a sharp object will pierce into tissue at a penetration pressure several times lower than that of a blunt object. Penetration by a blunt object, in contrast, results in a column of compressed material at the bottom of the wound created. Sharp-headed screwdrivers tended to follow the mode I fracture pattern, with wedging of the skin, whereas the straight-headed screwdriver resulted in a clearly defined skin plug (Fig. 4.5). In a similar vein, Parmar and his co-workers (2012) reported that there was a direct correlation between the cross-sectional area of a screwdriver head and the amount of force needed for penetration.

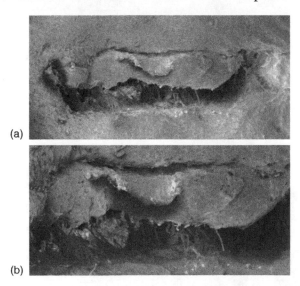

(a)

(b)

Figure 4.5 Scanning electron micrograph of an experimental penetrating injury by a straight head screwdriver into pig skin. Note the compressed tissue plug at the base of the wound (a). High-power view shows associated pullout collagen bundle bridges on the wound edges (b).

4.6 Blunt force trauma

As we have seen, skin consists essentially of a three-dimensional arrangement of collagen fibres. Its tensile strength depends primarily on fibre bundle size and cross-linking within this network. Fibre bundles have been shown to fracture in three principal ways (Arumugam *et al.*, 1994): firstly, they can fracture smoothly in a single plane perpendicular to the bundle's long axis; secondly, they can split down the long axis of the bundle and then progress to step-like perpendicular fractures; or, thirdly, they can fracture at right angles with fracture sites characterised by a brush-like pullout appearance (Fig. 4.6).

Blunt force trauma is often important evidence in cases of child or elder abuse, domestic violence and motor vehicle accidents. However, little is known of the relationship between visual appearance of such injuries and their causation. Whereas sharp force or high-speed trauma results in immediately visible injury, blunt trauma can result in deep muscular or subcutaneous disruption, without visible damage to the skin (Randeberg *et al.*, 2007). Evaluation based on visual inspection of such injuries is difficult and has been criticised for being both subjective and unreliable (Altemeier, 2001; Hornor, 2005). However, in criminal cases, having established expert evidence under Frye or Daubert standards, conclusions reached by experts are not typically evaluated in the light of the latest scientific research. As a consequence, a specialist witness overstating the evidence based on personal empirical experience is often not exposed by cross-examination. In criminal cases the defence is typically an unarmed adversary, often burdened with one-sided presentation of forensic evidence by the

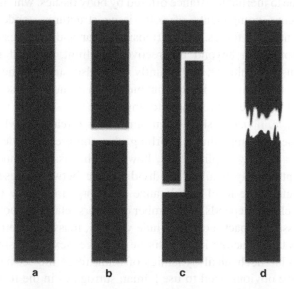

Figure 4.6 Three principal fracture mechanisms for a bundle of collagen fibres (a): smooth transverse fracture (b); stepped axial fracture (c); pullout fracture (d).

prosecution (Garrett and Neufeld, 2009). This is a problem in the case of blunt trauma, where visual examination has to be relied upon to determine the cause and nature of such injury. Moreover, the currently accepted scale of assessment of force applied (mild, moderate, considerable or severe) is not only highly subjective, but arbitrary and restrictive (Sharkey *et al.*, 2011).

What we do know, is that impact to the body results in some degree of deformation that can result in damage when it exceeds the tissue's recoverable limit. When the impacting object is either sharp, such as a knife or a screwdriver, or a high-speed projectile such as a bullet or missile, penetration injury typically results. This is simply because the energy of impact is concentrated on a small target area and, thus, there is little or no dissipation of energy (DiMaio, 1981). In contrast, when the impacting body is blunt, or the body strikes a blunt object at lower speed, the impact force is distributed over a larger area. Energy is dissipated and the severity of the penetration is reduced.

While sharp force injury is thus reasonably straightforward, blunt force injury is a more complex phenomenon and, hence, less well understood. For instance, not only will blunt force deform the target site, it will also initiate the propagation of stresses and strains within the tissue impacted. Depending on loading rates, geometry and material properties, tissue damage may result from shock waves, shearing or crushing of underlying tissue (Shen *et al.*, 2008). Injury caused by an impacting object is related to a number of factors, including the energy delivered at impact, the shape and size of the object and the properties of the area impacted. In one of the earlier analyses of blunt force trauma, Viano *et al.* (1989) suggested that damage was primarily due to inertial resistance offered by body tissues, which, together with elastic and viscous components of soft tissue structures, tended to generate traumatic deformational forces. Strain (tensile, shear and compressive), resulting from tissue deformation beyond the recoverable limit, resulted in lacerations, ruptures and crushing injuries. Importantly, they also stressed the role of strain rate on the generation of injury. Recall that biological tissues are viscoelastic, which means that their tolerance and response to impact are rate sensitive (Viano and Lau, 1988). For instance, if one pushes down onto one's forearm slowly, the skin and underlying tissue deforms, thus absorbing the compressional energy without damage. Under a rapidly applied load, however, the tissues cannot deform fast enough, and rupture may result. The dividing line between these is the injury threshold and defines the level of tolerance of an organ or tissue to impact. The injury threshold clearly depends on a number of factors relating to both the impactor and the target tissue. Impact factors include velocity, mass, geometry and angle of impact; whereas target factors include tissue site, age, sex, body size and disease.

Research into biomechanical dynamics of blunt force impact has always been constrained by the obvious need to use human surrogates in the form of cadavers, live or dead experimental animals, or mechanical models. One such model is that of Whittle *et al.* (2008), who used a drop-tube setup and a target tissue made of hydrated, open-celled foam to which a silicone skin simulant had been fused. What they found was that, on initial impact, the water-filled foam acted as a rigid body because of the incompressibility of water directly beneath the contact area. This resulted in the skin becoming highly compressed and squeezed between the impacting body and the underlying foam (Fig. 4.7). As the strain rate increased, underlying water-filled cells fractured when the tensile strain in the cell walls became sufficiently high, resulting in subsurface rupture. Importantly, they showed that, while nearly all impacts resulted in subsurface rupture, skin laceration occurred in fewer than half of the impacts. This suggested that, during blunt force impact, tissue injury progresses from the inside out, which is the opposite to sharp force injury, which progresses from the outside in.

In an effort to understand the pathophysiological nature of head lacerations caused by blunt force trauma, Sharkey *et al.* (2011) devised an experimental drop-tower experiment to assess the biomechanical aspects of blunt force trauma to the head, using domestic pig heads. Their test rig was designed to deliver perpendicular blows of measurable force by four impactors: a hammer, broom handle, a training shoe and a piece of wooden flooring. While the patterns of skin laceration varied considerably, they did find that the minimum force required to generate a laceration (i.e. the injury threshold) was at least 4 kN, which accorded with Whittle's calculations of a range between 2 kN and 10 kN. Predictably, implements that focus impact (hammer, broom handle) resulted in more severe laceration than those

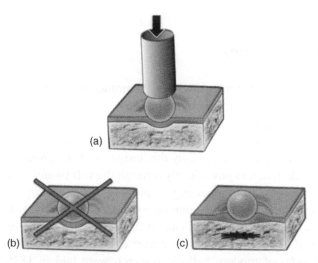

(a)

(b)   (c)

Figure 4.7 Blunt force injury modelled with a drop-tube setup (a) that delivers a known shape with a known weight from an adjustable height. At impact, the dermal tissue is not evenly stretched (b); rather, it is disproportionally stretched directly beneath the impactor (c). Subdermal tissue is more hydrostatic, and tends to rupture before the dermal tissue, giving rise to bruising. Hence, in blunt force injury to soft tissue, wounding progresses from the inside out.

that disperse impact, such as a shoe. The question now arises: will a round shape penetrate skin easier than an edged shape?

As we have seen, Shergold and Fleck (2004) have shown that a sharp indenter penetrates more easily than a blunt one. Hence, it seems intuitive that an edged implement will penetrate more easily than a rounded one. Examining this issue, Freeman and Lemen (2006) found it useful to separate initial penetration into two different processes: firstly, crack propagation; and, secondly, tissue deformation. Crack initiation requires enough energy to fracture all the chemical bonds in the area of impact, and hence, the injury threshold (fracture energy) is the minimum amount of energy required to fracture the skin at the site of impact. Again, intuitively, one would expect that the fracture energy is strongly related to the strength of the chemical bonds holding the skin together. This, however, is a misconception (Gordon, 2003). In fact, differences in chemical bond strengths among materials are insignificant when compared to the massive differences in fracture energy between brittle and tough substances. In brittle substances, shallow depth of deformation enables most energy to be directed at breaking chemical bonds along the fracture path. In contrast, tough materials absorb impact energy through deformation before cracks are initiated. This is exactly how tough materials, such as skin, resist crack propagation. A round-shaped impacting object first deforms and then tears the skin; whereas an angled object can concentrate energy at the site of impact, thus initiating and propagating the crack before it deforms the skin away from the rupture.

4.7   Ballistic trauma

Scientists still do not fully understand how the immense energy involved in ballistic impact translates into soft tissue injury. Clearly work and energy, together with force, velocity and momentum play important roles, but these are confounded by additional aspects such as angle of impact and shape of the projectile. Added to these factors are those incorporated by the designers of the projectiles themselves; while some are designed to pass cleanly through the soft tissues, others are created for the specific purpose of fragmenting or spinning within the target. Scientists who study ballistic trauma are now beginning to understand how soft tissues, such as skin, behave under ballistic impact. One of the best books on the subject is that of Kneubuehl *et al.* (2011), to which the reader is strongly directed.

The foundations of modern ballistic research were laid in 1875 by the Swiss physician Emil Theodor Kocher (1841–1917), who attempted to formulate the explosive wounding effects of small calibre rifles. The view at the time was that bullets caused soft tissue damage by one of three mechanisms: melting of the bullet on impact, hydraulic pressure, or centrifugal forces created by the spinning projectile. Kocher noticed that neither partial melting nor centrifugal force were significant drivers of tissue damage. It also became clear that, in addition to velocity, the mass, shape and construction of the bullet were critically important to the wounding process. Using observations on shots fired into a series of targets, ranging from moist clay, cans and soap blocks, to containers filled with water or gelatin, Kocher made sense of wounding mechanisms by suggesting that there were four elements to the explosive loss of kinetic energy at the target site. Firstly, he argued that a small amount of energy was converted into heat; secondly, some kinetic energy drove the soft tissue along the bullet path away perpendicularly, thereby creating a temporary cavity; thirdly, energy was used in crushing the tissue ahead of the bullet, thus carving a bullet tract; and finally, kinetic energy deformed the bullet itself (Fackler and Dougherty, 1991).

Alarmed by the wounds inflicted on soldiers at the start of the Second World War, the United States Government funded a Wound Ballistics Research Group (WBRG) at Princeton University under the leadership of the physiologist E. Newton Harvey and the anatomist, Elmer Butler. The WBRG was charged with the quantitative study of ballistic wounding of different projectile shapes, masses and velocities, so that maximum incapacitation could be predicted. Because they realised that when a projectile strikes, most of its effects are over in a few milliseconds, the WBRG decided to use techniques that could register what happened in a ten-thousandth, or even a millionth of a second (Harvey, 1948). Using then state-of-the-art oscilloscopes, high speed cameras, micro-second radiography and piezoelectric crystals, the group sought to define a 'standard wound' created by a round ball fired into water, plasticine and living animals. What they found was this: when an eighth-inch (3 mm) ball bearing was fired at a cat's thigh at 3000 ft/s (914 m/s), with energy of about 3.7×10^8 ergs (37 J), sharp, high-pressure pulses or shockwaves were initiated that radiated from the point of impact with a period of three micro-seconds, at maximum pressures of 170 lbs/sq inch (1.17 MPa) (Harvey and McMillen, 1947). Once it penetrated the skin, the bearing pulverised the tissue in front of it, spattering debris out of both the entrance and exit holes. Then came their crucial observation: the bullet lost about 85% of its energy during passage, from which they calculated a retardation equation:

$$R = dv/dt = av^2$$

also known as the velocity squared law, where the velocity is v, and a is the retardation coefficient. The retardation coefficient was related to characteristics of both the projectile and its target tissue, where:

$$a = C_D \rho A / 2m$$

and C_D is the drag coefficient (for muscle, 0.450), ρ is the density of the medium, A the cross-sectional area of the missile and m is the mass of the missile (Harvey, 1948).

Importantly, energy lost was due mostly to a large and explosively expanding temporary cavity that pulsated at a diminishing rhythm of about three milliseconds before collapsing into a permanent wound shot channel. The temporary cavity had the ability to destroy at a distance – muscle fibres, nerves and vessels were violently ripped apart, and bones were fractured by the radially expanding cavity.

We have already introduced the concept of temporary cavity formation (Chapter 3). Essentially, some of the bullet's kinetic energy is used to rip the tissue apart, which forms the wound tract, and some energy is transferred from the projectile to accelerate the surrounding soft tissue radially away from the bullet tract. In other words, as it traverses soft tissue, the bullet creates a shot path as well as a hollow space behind it. For a given bullet size and velocity, the size of this space (the temporary cavity envelope) depends on the elasticity of the soft tissue. The smaller the Young's modulus, the larger the cavity. This is simply because the forces tending to restore the deflected tissue are relatively smaller. Immediately after the passage of the bullet, its kinetic energy having been converted to elastic energy, the temporary cavity subsides until all the remaining elastic energy is dissipated. Clinically, Kneubuehl *et al.* (2011) have divided the envelope of damage caused by temporary cavitation into three zones (Fig. 4.8).

Zone 1 is the area of permanent tissue destruction caused by the expanding temporary cavity. This is not to be confused with the shot path, which is the channel of destruction caused by the bullet itself, and, hence, Zone 1 is not a tube of the same diameter as the bullet.

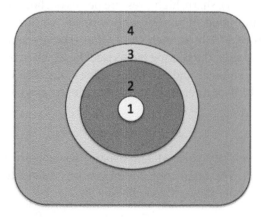

Figure 4.8 Diagrammatic representation of the damage zones resulting from the explosive formation of a temporary cavity in soft tissue. 1: Zone of destruction. 2: Zone of extravasation. 3: Zone of expansion of the temporary cavity. 4: Tissue unaffected by the temporary cavitation. (Adapted from Kneubuehl *et al.*, 2011.)

Zone 2 consists of an area of blood seepage into tissue that was stretched but not permanently damaged.

Zone 3 is the area of expansion of the temporary cavity, where tissue is stretched, but otherwise unaffected. In other words, the total envelope of the temporary cavity.

As mentioned before, a distinctive and important feature of the impact of a bullet on soft tissue is the hydrostatic shock waves it may or may not create, and their effect on the tissue beyond the reach of the temporary cavity. This is a contentious issue, with some authors seeing the phenomenon as a myth, and others as gospel (see, for instance, Jandial *et al.*, 2008, versus Courtney and Courtney, 2011). Again, it was Harvey and McMillen (1947) who conducted the first experimental studies of the relationship between ballistic waves and tissue damage. They measured these ultra-fast pressure transients using piezoelectrical pressure transducers and spark shadowgraph photography, and concluded that observed injury caused by the transient pressure waves was associated with gas pockets in the body, such as the lungs.

Unfortunately, this left us with a large grey area. Hunters know that game animals can be incapacitated instantly, without the bullet disrupting vital organs. Similarly, descriptions of rifle wounds received during the Vietnam War include references to abdominal injury, broken bones and neurological disruption from peripheral flesh wounds (Courtney and Courtney, 2011). The obvious question that now emerges is: could this damage be due to the remote effects of a rapid pressure pulse caused by the bullet? Although there does not appear to be a definitive answer, studies by Suneson and his co-workers (1987, 1988, 1990a,b), and Wang *et al.* (2004) provide some evidence for central neurological damage caused by high-energy oscillating pressure waves from peripheral bullet impacts in experimental animals. This has given rise to the hypothesis that ballistic injury can result independently of the wounding caused by the crushing effects of the rapidly expanding temporary cavity. A shock wave has been described as a form of acoustic wave caused by a single, abrupt and highly intense excitation, with its damage potential residing in the sudden changes between positive and negative pressure amplitudes in relation to the resting pressure (Kneubuehl *et al.*, 2011).

There is another point of interest in this brief discussion of pressure waves: namely the pathophysiological consequences of such waves on distant tissues. A shock wave is an enormous, yet solitary event, with the wavefront radiating outwards from the point of impact. Heterogeneity of bodily tissues ensures that the wave undergoes consequential deflection, scatter and absorption. In reviewing the relevant literature, Kneubuehl *et al.* (2011) conclude that it is not the pressure itself that causes tissue damage, but rather the rapid increase followed by decrease in pressure, as biological tissues can only be injured by stretching or shear, and not by compression. The bottom line is that research into damage caused by ballistic impact has not kept pace with the inventiveness of the designers of arms, ammunition and improvised explosive devices.

4.8 Bitemarks

As we have seen, the biomechanical properties of skin are highly complex, being governed not only by its geometry, anatomy or the interaction of collagen and elastin networks, but also by factors such as cleavage lines, age, sex and health. Two fundamental tenets underlie the interpretation of bitemarks: firstly, that the human anterior dentition is unique; and, secondly, that this individuality is accurately reflected by the bitemark (Kieser *et al.*, 2007). The mechanical behaviour of the epidermis and dermis largely determines how a bite will be reflected as a skin wound. At its simplest level, the forces applied to the skin during biting result in compression, tension and shear (Fig. 4.9).

In a series of papers, Bush and her colleagues have investigated the biomechanical confounders of bitemark analysis (Miller *et al.*, 2009; Bush *et al.*, 2009, 2010). These highlighted the role of Langer's lines; bites perpendicular to the cleavage line shift the stress/strain curve to the left, which means skin becomes stiffer more rapidly (Fig. 4.10). Bites that cross Langer's lines may therefore distort unevenly; in fact it is hard to see how the same dentition can create consistently similar bite patterns on the same victim. They concluded that, while the dentition can be accurately measured and

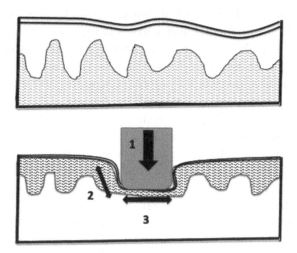

Figure 4.9 Basic force transmissions during biting of the skin. The striking tooth generates compression (1), shear (2) and tension (3).

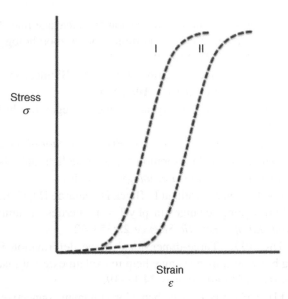

Figure 4.10 Idealised stress/strain curve for bitemark impression on skin; bites across Langer's lines (I) will encounter stiffer, less elastic tissue than those along cleavage lines (II). This may result in significant bitemark distortion.

described during bitemark analysis, its imprint on the skin does not yield reproducible results. In short, the skin is a poor impression material.

References

Altemeier WA. 2001. Interpreting bruises in children. *Pediatric Annals* **30**:517–20.

Arumugam V, Naresh MD, Sanjeevi R. 1994. Effect of strain rate on fracture behavior of skin. *Journal of Biosciences* **19**:307–13.

Boyer G, Laquieze L, LeBot A, Laquiese S, Zahouani H. 2009. Dynamic indentation on human skin in vivo: ageing effects. *Skin Research and Technology* **15**:55–67.

Briggaman RA. 1982. Biochemical composition of the epidermal-dermal junction and other basement membrane. *Journal of Investigative Dermatology* **78**:1–6.

Bush J, Fergusom MW, Mason T, McGrouther G. 2007. The dynamic rotation of Langer's lines on facial expression. *Journal of Plastic Reconstructive and Aesthetic Surgery* **60**:393–9.

Bush MA, Miller RG, Bush PJ, Dorion RBJ. 2009. Biomechanical factors in human dermal bitemarks in a cadaver model. *Journal of Forensic Sciences* **54**:167–76.

Bush MA, Cooper HI, Dorion RBJ. 2010. Inquiry into the scientific basis for bitemark profiling and arbitrary distortion compensation. *Journal of Forensic Sciences* **55**:976–83.

Byard RW, Gehl A, Tsokos M. 2005. Skin tension and cleavage lines (Langer's lines) causing distortion of ante- and postmortem wound morphology. *International Journal of Legal Medicine* **119**:226–30.

Chadwick EKJ, Nicol AC, Lane JV, Gray TGF. 1999. Biomechanics of knife stab attacks. *Forensic Science International* **105**:35–44.

Courtney M, Courtney A. 2011. History and evidence regarding hydrostatic shock. *Neurosurgery* **68**:E596–8.

Cox HT. 1941. The cleavage lines of the skin. *British Journal of Surgery* **29**:234–40.

DiMaio VJ. 1981. Penetration and perforation of skin by bullets and missiles. *American Journal of Forensic Medicine and Pathology* **2**:107–10.

Diridollou S, Vabre V, Berson M, Vaillant L, Black D, Lagarde JM, Gregoire JM, Gall Y, Patat F. 2001. Skin ageing: changes in physical properties of human skin *in vivo*. *International Journal of Cosmetic Science* **23**:353–62.

Dodd KT, Gross DR. 1991. Three-dimensional tissue deformation in subcutaneous tissue overlying bony prominences may help to explain external load transfer to the interstitium. *Journal of Biomechanics* **24**:11–19.

Dunn MG, Silver FH. 1983. Viscoelastic behavior of human connective tissues: relative contributions of viscous and elastic components. *Connective Tissue Research* **12**:59–70.

Escoffier C, DeRigal J, Rochefort A, Vasselet R, Leveque JL, Agache PG. 1980. Age-related mechanical properties of human skin: an *in vivo* study. *Journal of Investigative Dermatology* **93**:353–7.

Fackler ML, Dougherty PJ. 1991. Theodor Kocher and the scientific foundation of wound ballistics. *Surgery* **172**:153–60.

Freeman PW, Lemen C. 2006. Puncturing ability of idealised canine teeth: edged and non-edged shanks. *Journal of Zoology* **269**:51–6.

Garrett BL, Neufeld PJ. 2009. Invalid forensic science testimony and wrongful convictions. *Virginia Law Review* **95**:1–97.

Gibson T. 1978. Karl Langer and his lines. *British Journal of Plastic Surgery* **31**:1–2.

Gibson T, Kenedi RM, Craik JE. 1965. The mobile micro-architecture of dermal collagen. *British Journal of Surgery* **52**:764–70.

Gordon JE. 2003. *Structures, or Why Things Don't Fall Down*, 2nd Edition. Da Capo Press, Cambridge, MA.

Green MA. 1978. Stab wound dynamics – a recording technique for use in medicolegal investigations. *Journal of the Forensic Science Society* **18**:161–3.

Harvey EN. 1948. The mechanism of wounding by high velocity missiles. *Proceedings of the American Philosophical Society* **92**:294–304.

Harvey EN, McMillen JH. 1947. An experimental study of shock waves resulting from the impact of high velocity missiles on animal tissues. *Journal of Experimental Medicine* **85**:321–8.

Hornor G. 2005. Physical abuse: recognition and reporting. *Journal of Paediatric Health Care* **19**:4–11.

Jandial R, Reichwage B, Levy M, Duenas V, Sturdivan L. 2008. Ballistics for the neurosurgeon. *Neurosurgery* **62**:472–80.

Jones S, Nokes L, Leadbetter S. 1994. The mechanics of stab wounding. *Forensic Science International* **67**:59–63.

Kendall K, Fuller KNG. 1987. J-shaped stress/strain curves and crack resistance of biological materials. *Journal of Physics D: Applied Physics* **20**:1596–1600.

Kieser JA, Bernal V, Waddell JN, Raju S. 2007. The uniqueness of the human anterior dentition: a geometric morphometric analysis. *Journal of Forensic Sciences* **52**:671–7.

Kieser JA, Whittle K, Wong B, Waddell JN, Ichim I, Swain M, Taylor M, Nicholson H. 2008a. Understanding craniofacial blunt force injury: a biomechanical perspective. *Forensic Pathology Reviews* **5**:37–51.

Kieser JA, Bernal V, Gonzalez P, Birch W, Turmaine M, Ichim I. 2008b. Analysis of experimental cranial wounding from screwdriver trauma. *International Journal of Legal Medicine* **122**:179–87.

Kneubuehl BP, Coupland RM, Rothchild MA, Thali MJ. 2011. *Wound Ballistics*. Springer, Berlin.

Knight B. 1975. The dynamics of stab wounds. *Forensic Science* **6**:249–55.

Langer AK. 1861. Zur Anatomie und Physiologie der Haut. I. Über die Spaltbarkeit der Cutis. *Sitzungberichte der Akademie der Wissenschaften* **44**:19–46.

Langer K. 1978a. On the anatomy and physiology of skin I. *British Journal of Plastic Surgery* **31**:3–8.

Langer K. 1978b. On the anatomy and physiology of skin II. *British Journal of Plastic Surgery* **31**:93–106.

Langer K. 1978c. On the anatomy and physiology of skin III. *British Journal of Plastic Surgery* **31**:185–99.

Lavker RM, Zheng PS, Dong G. 1986. Morphology of aged skin. *Dermatology Clinics* **4**:379–89.

Le KM, Madsen BL, Barth PW, Ksander GA, Angell JB, Vistnes LM. 1984. An in-depth look at pressure sores using monolithic silicon pressure sensors. *Plastic and Reconstructive Surgery* **74**:745–54.

Miller RG, Bush PJ, Dorion RBJ, Bush MA. 2009. Uniqueness of the dentition as impressed in human skin: a cadaver model. *Journal of Forensic Sciences* **54**:909–14.

Montagna W, Parakkal PF. 1974. *The Structure and Function of Skin*. Academic Press, New York.

O'Callaghan PT, Jones MD, James DS, Leadbeatter S, Holt CA, Nokes LDM. 1999. Dynamics of stab wounds: force required for penetration of various cadaveric human tissues. *Forensic Science International* **104**:173–8.

Oxlund H, Manscot J, Vidiik A. 1988. The role of elastin in the mechanical properties of skin. *Journal of Biomechanics* **21**:213–18.

Parmar K, Hainsworth SV, Rutty GN. 2012. Quantification of forces required for stabbing with screwdrivers and other blunter instruments. *International Journal of Legal Medicine* **126**:43–53. doi:10.1007/s00414-011-0562-9.

Pasyk KA, Thomas SV, Hassett CA, Cherry GW, Faller R. 1989. Regional differences in capillary density of the normal human dermis. *Plastic and Reconstructive Surgery* **83**:939–47.

Payne PA. 1991. Measurement of properties and function of skin. *Clinical Physics and Physiological Measurement* **12**:105–29.

Randeberg LL, Winnem AM, Langlois NE, Larsen ELP, Haaverstad R, Skallerud B, Haugen OA, Svaasand H. 2007. Skin changes following minor trauma. *Lasers in Surgery and Medicine* **39**:403–13.

Rawlins AV. 2006. Ethnic skin types: are there differences in skin structure and function? *International Journal of Cosmetic Science* **28**:79–93.

Richey M, Richey HK, Fenske NA. 1988. Aging-related skin changes: development and clinical meaning. *Geriatrics* **43**:49–64.

Ridge MD, Wright V. 1966. The directional effects of skin. A bioengineering study of skin with particular reference to Langer's lines. *Journal of Investigative Dermatology* **46**:341–6.

Sanders JE, Goldstein BS, Leotta DF. 1995. Skin response to mechanical stress: adaptation rather than breakdown – a review of the literature. *Journal of Rehabilitation Research and Development* **32**:214–26.

Saukko P, Knight B. 2004. *Knight's Forensic Pathology*, 3rd Edition. Hodder Arnold, London.

Sharkey EJ, Cassidy M, Brady J, Gilchrist MD, NicDaeid N. 2011. Investigation of the force associated with the formation of lacerations and skull fractures. *International Journal of Legal Medicine*. doi:10.1007/s00414-011-0608-z.

Shen W, Niu Y, Mattrey RF, Fournier A, Corbeil A, Kono Y. 2008. Development and validation of subject-specific finite element models for blunt trauma study. *Journal of Biomechanical Engineering* **130**:1–13.

Shergold OA, Fleck NA. 2004. Mechanism of deep penetration of soft solids, with application to the injection and wounding of skin. *Proceedings of the Royal Society A Mathematics, Physics and Engineering Sciences* **460**:3037–58.

Shuster S, Black MM, McVitie E. 1975. The influence of age and sex on skin thickness. *British Journal of Dermatology* **93**:639–43.

Silver FH, Freeman JW, DeVore D. 2001a. Viscoelastic properties of human skin and processed dermis. *Skin Research and Technology* **7**:16–23.

Silver FH, Christiansen DL, Snowhill PB, Chen Y. 2001b. Transition from viscous to elastic-dependency of mechanical properties of self-assembled collagen fibres. *Journal of Applied Polymer Science* **79**:134–42.

Silver FH, Seehra GP, Freeman JW, DeVore D. 2002. Viscoelastic properties of young and old human dermis: a proposed molecular mechanism for elastic energy storage in collagen and elastin. *Journal of Applied Polymer Science* **86**:1978–85.

Suneson A, Hansson HA, Seeman T. 1987. Peripheral high-energy missile hits cause pressure changes and damage to the nervous system: experimental studies on pigs. *Journal of Trauma* **27**:782–9.

Suneson A, Hansson HA, Seeman T. 1988. Central and peripheral nervous damage following high-energy missile wounds in the thigh. *Journal of Trauma* **28**: S197–203.

Suneson A, Hansson HA, Seeman T. 1990a. Pressure wave injuries to the nervous system caused by high-energy missile extremity impact I: light and electron microscopic study on pigs. *Journal of Trauma* **30**:281–97.

Suneson A, Hansson HA, Seeman T. 1990b. Pressure wave injuries to the nervous system caused by high-energy missile extremity impact II: distant effects on the central nervous system. *Journal of Trauma* **30**:295–306.

Takema Y, Yorimoto Y, Kawai M, Imokawa G. 1994. Age-related changes in the elastic properties and thickness of human facial skin. *British Journal of Dermatology* **131**:641–8.

Viano DC, Lau IV. 1988. A viscous tolerance criterion for soft tissue injury assessment. *Journal of Biomechanics* **21**:387–99.

Viano DC, King AI, Melvin JW, Weber K. 1989. Injury biomechanics research: an essential element in the prevention of trauma. *Journal of Biomechanics* **22**:403–17.

Wang Q, Wang Z, Zhu P, Jiang J. 2004. Alterations of the myelin basic protein and ultrastructure in the limbic system and the early stage of trauma-related stress disorder in dogs. *Journal of Trauma* **56**:604–10.

Whittle K, Kieser, JA, Ichim I, Swain MV, Waddell JN, Livingstone V, Taylor M. 2008. The biomechanical modeling of non-ballistic skin wounding: blunt force injury. *Forensic Science, Medicine, and Pathology* **4**:33–9.

5

The mechanics of bloodstain pattern formation

Mark Jermy and Michael Taylor

5.1   Introduction to bloodstain pattern analysis

Bloodstain Pattern Analysis (BPA) is the study of bloodstains to extract information about what occurred at a bloodletting event. DNA profiling can help identify the wounded person and, in some cases, a body part from which the blood originated. BPA can yield information on the positions of the victim and assailant, the type of weapon, and subsequent motions of the participants. One of the first steps in analysing any bloodstained scene is the classification of the bloodstain patterns in it. Bloodstain patterns can be classified into broad groups. *Transfer patterns* are formed by a bloodied object coming into contact with a surface and perhaps being subsequently transferred onto other surfaces, for example by footprint. *Drip patterns* are formed by blood gathering on a surface under gravity and dripping onto lower surfaces. *Spatter patterns* are caused by blood being broken up into droplets, which are dispersed through the air and land on nearby surfaces. The size and shape of spatter stains can yield information on the position of origin of the blood and, hence, important information about the locations and actions of the participants.

The Bloodstain Pattern Analyst attempts to solve an 'inverse problem'. Starting from the bloodstain pattern observed at a crime scene, the analyst desires to work back to a probable wounding event. This is a difficult task, because there is often more than one wounding event that can lead to a particular bloodstain pattern. The body of knowledge on how these ambiguities can be resolved, and when they cannot, is beyond this text, but has been developed by a community of experienced individuals (the Scientific Working Group On Bloodstain Pattern Analysis (SWGSTAIN): www.swgstain.org; the International Association of Bloodstain Pattern Analysts (IABPA): www.iabpa.org), with some of this knowledge described in the standard texts (e.g. James *et al.*, 2005; Bevel and Gardner, 2008). This chapter describes the 'forward problem': the physical processes which occur between the release of blood and the formation of the stain pattern. An understanding of these processes is essential to the solution of the inverse problem and to defining limits on the probability of the conclusions drawn.

When it comes to achieving a reliable classification of a bloodstain pattern, an understanding of the dynamic processes that occur during its formation is invaluable. The mechanics of blood as a liquid and its behaviour during the

Forensic Biomechanics, First Edition. Jules Kieser, Michael Taylor and Debra Carr.
© 2013 John Wiley & Sons, Ltd. Published 2013 by John Wiley & Sons, Ltd.

formation of common spatter patterns is the subject of this chapter. The discussion that follows is based solidly on the principles of fluid mechanics and draws on examples from a recent comprehensive study of bloodstain pattern formation using high-speed video imaging (Laber *et al.*, 2008). We begin with some basic definitions and then follow the formation stages of a spatter pattern from its origin in some liquid breakup event which results in the formation of droplets, the subsequent projection of these drops through the air and their final impact on a surface to form the bloodstain pattern.

Basics of fluid mechanics

The term 'fluid' is often used to mean a liquid, but in fact includes both liquids and gases. These are states of matter which will deform to fill a container and which cannot support a shear stress without moving.

In gases, the molecules are far apart and they generally experience mild attractive forces that attempt to move them closer together, reducing their energy (Fig. 5.1). Due to these forces and random thermal motion, gas molecules occasionally approach each other closely. Molecules that are very close together have high positive intermolecular energy and thus experience repulsive forces that cause them to veer away from one another. This interaction is called a collision.

In liquids, the molecules lie between these two extremes: close together, but not too close, with low intermolecular energy and attractive or cohesive forces, bringing them closer together until a mild collision separates them again.

Blood is a liquid, and liquids are virtually incompressible. If one took a bicycle pump, filled it with air, sealed the opening and pushed on the plunger, it would require some force to compress the air, but it would be possible to reduce its volume

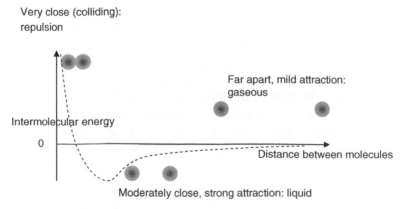

Figure 5.1 The force and energy between molecules depends on the distance between them.

considerably. If the pump were filled with water it would require excessive force to move the plunger, and in fact the pump would probably leak or burst before the volume of the water was reduced more than a fraction of 1%.

The deep-diving submersible bathyscaphe (submarine) 'Trieste' is an example of the incompressibility of liquids. It was used to descend to the bottom of the Mariana Trench, near Guam, which at approximately 11 km deep is the deepest known point in the ocean. The crew were housed in a spherical steel compartment with walls 12.7 cm thick. All submersibles have a buoyancy tank filled with something less dense than water. In most submersibles this is compressed air, but, at the depths the Trieste dived to, an air-filled vessel would have imploded due to the immense seawater pressure, unless the walls were so thick that the tank could not be made buoyant. Instead of air, the buoyancy tank in the bathyscaphe was filled with petrol (gasoline), which, being incompressible, prevented the tank from imploding. The density of petrol being less than water, the craft had positive buoyancy when the ballast was dropped.

The laws of Newtonian physics, described in Chapter 1, apply to fluids, except if they are moving at near the speed of light, or experiencing nuclear reactions – neither of which apply to BPA. Some other physical principles can be applied to predict how fluids will behave. Energy is conserved: the total amount of energy is the same, although it can be converted from one form to another. For example, a droplet thrown up through the air loses kinetic energy, but gains gravitational potential energy; through air resistance (drag), a small amount of its kinetic energy is also converted to heat in the surrounding air (Fig. 5.2). A droplet impacting on a surface changes shape, losing kinetic energy and gaining surface energy, an energy associated with surface tension.

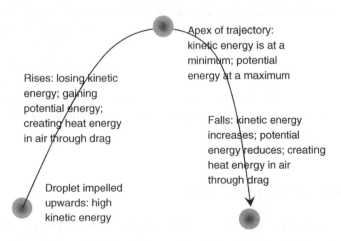

Figure 5.2 Energy is converted from one form to another during the flight of a droplet. The total energy in the droplet plus the total energy in the air remains the same.

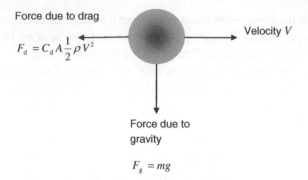

$$F_d = C_d A \frac{1}{2} \rho V^2$$

Force due to drag

Velocity V

Force due to gravity

$$F_g = mg$$

Figure 5.3 Forces on a droplet moving through the air.

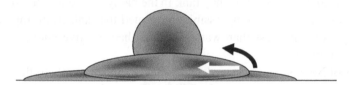

Figure 5.4 A droplet strikes a solid surface and spreads. In the spreading mantle of blood, viscous shear forces slow the spread (white arrow). On the surface, surface tension forces also slow the spread (black arrow).

Momentum is conserved, meaning that the momentum possessed by any given mass of fluid will remain the same unless it is acted on by an external force. A falling droplet is acted on by gravity and drag and changes its velocity (Fig. 5.3). A mass of blood spreading over a surface is acted on by surface tension and viscous forces which slow its spread (Fig. 5.4).

Mass is also conserved, and this proves a useful basis for writing formulae to describe fluid motion, keeping track of the fluid passing into and out of a fixed region of space. If a stream of blood flowing across the surface slows down as it gets further from the source, the stream must become wider or deeper.

Another physical principle has proved useful in fluid mechanics: disorder (entropy) increases with time in any system unless work is done to reduce it, in which case entropy increases in the system doing the work. It requires effort to keep a desk tidy, which results in the generation of heat in the one doing the tidying, and this heat is a form of disorder.

5.2   Forces acting on fluids

The important forces that determine the behaviour of blood released in a wounding event are gravity, arterial pressure, surface tension, viscosity and aerodynamic drag.

Gravity

Gravity is the simplest, exerting a force vertically downwards with a magnitude equal to the mass of the blood m multiplied by the acceleration due to gravity g:

$$F_{gravity} = mg$$

The exact value of g varies slightly from place to place with altitude and the density of nearby rocks, but $9.81\,m/s^2$ is sufficiently accurate for calculation in most biomechanics problems. Multiplying the mass in kilograms by g in metres per second squared gives a value of force, $F_{gravity}$, in newtons, the standard SI unit of force. This force is properly called the weight, which should be measured in newtons, where the mass is measured in kilograms.

Arterial pressure

Arterial blood pressure in a healthy human adult varies from 90 to 100 mmHg or 9.3–13 kPa above atmospheric pressure, varying of course as the heart beats. This difference between this pressure and atmospheric pressure is important in the projection of blood when an artery is pierced. The pressure in the jet of blood drops to atmospheric pressure almost as soon as the blood leaves the wound, but the momentum imparted by the pressure difference can carry the jet some metres in an arcing trajectory as gravity accelerates the blood towards the ground.

Surface tension

Surface tension refers to both a force and a characteristic of a liquid, like density or viscosity. The surface tension forces only arise at the interface between the liquid and some other substance; for example the surface between a liquid and air, or liquid and its own vapour (e.g. water and steam), or the interface between two liquids which cannot mix (e.g. water and oil). A force of similar origins, but properly called interfacial tension, arises at the interface of a liquid and a solid, or a gas and a solid, or two different solids.

These forces arise because of the energy stored in the interaction between molecules. Generally speaking, molecules experience attractive forces if far apart, so reduce their energy by moving closer together, as seen in liquids. There is some limit to how close they can approach one another; nearer than this, strong repulsive forces push them apart again (Fig. 5.1).

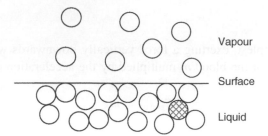

Figure 5.5 Molecules in the bulk liquid, and near the liquid–air interface.

Now consider a molecule on the surface of a liquid droplet (Fig. 5.5). On one side it has other molecules closely crowded, as in a liquid, with low energy. On the other side the nearest molecules are much further away and the energy is higher. So molecules on the surface are in a higher energy state than those molecules deep inside the liquid that have close contact with like molecules on all sides. The surface, thus, has a higher energy than the bulk liquid. The surface tension value of the liquid (0.072 N/m for water at 20 °C) is a measure of this energy (as the units newtons of force per unit length, are identical to joules of energy per unit area). Like most physical systems, the droplet will spontaneously attempt to reduce its energy to a minimum. This it does by minimising the surface area. The surface energy gives rise to a force which pulls the drop into the shape which has the least surface energy.

For a free-falling drop, this shape is a sphere, which of all possible shapes has the smallest surface area for a given volume. For a stationary drop on a solid surface (a sessile drop), the lowest energy shape is lenticular (lens-like), because what is being minimised is the total of the liquid–air surface energy, the liquid–solid surface energy and the air–solid surface energy (Fig. 5.6). If the liquid–solid surface energy is very high, as it is for example with a droplet of water on a leaf or a feather, the drop will minimise the area of contact with the solid surface (minimise the area of the liquid–solid interface) and form a raised, near-spherical drop which rolls off the surface easily (Fig. 5.6a). Such solid surfaces are called hydrophobic (water hating) as they repel water. Plant leaves are hydrophobic, and rain or dew results in near-spherical water drops which roll off easily. On the other hand, a water droplet on a cotton surface will form a flat lens shape, with a larger water–solid surface area and

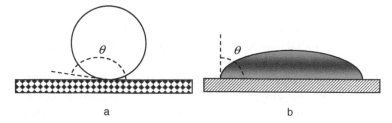

Figure 5.6 Sessile droplets with contact angle θ shown (a) on a hydrophobic (non-wetting) surface, and (b) on a hydrophilic (wettable) surface.

smaller water–air surface area (relative to the drop on a feather) (Fig. 5.6b). This is 'wetting' the surface. The solid surface in this case is hydrophilic (water loving) and 'wettable'. This is why cotton is a poor choice for waterproof garments, compared to a hydrophobic material like polar fleece or polyester.

The angle between the liquid–air interface and the liquid–solid interface, at the point where liquid, air and solid meet, is called the contact angle. The value of this angle is one way of characterising surface energies. For a stationary drop on a perfectly flat, level, solid surface, the contact angle takes a unique value determined by the energy per unit area of the liquid–air, liquid–solid and air–solid interfaces. The actual contact angle, however, is modified by roughness and dirt on the solid surface. It is the average of the angles made with a number of small protrusions on a rough surface, and dirt, especially oil and grease, that changes the surface energy. A droplet moving forwards over a surface will bulge over the point where liquid, solid and air meet to increase the contact angle. A droplet receding from the contact line will flatten and reduce the contact angle.

The property that is commonly referred to as surface tension for a liquid is the value of the surface energy per unit area of the liquid–air interface. It is often given the symbol σ. For pure water this is 0.072 N/m at 20 °C. It is altered by the presence of certain molecules dissolved in the liquid. Any molecule that modifies surface tension is called a surfactant. Detergents typically reduce the liquid–air surface energy. By changing the contact angle, addition of detergent will encourage a droplet to spread over the surface (wet the surface). Detergents also allow large bubbles to be produced, because in a bubble the internal air pressure, which is higher than atmospheric, is opposed by surface tension forces, in an equilibrium which results in a stable, hollow bubble.

Surface energy is a function of the radius of curvature of the surface. Figure 5.7b shows a drop with the equatorial or meridian plane drawn in. This is a plane that bisects the drop. If we slice the drop at this plane, we would find that there is a surface tension force at the edge of this plane pulling up, trying to minimise the surface area. The surface tension force is balanced in a drop by a pressure force. The air pressure inside the drop is actually greater than the atmospheric pressure outside. The excess pressure is denoted by Δp. The pressure force acting on this equatorial plane is Δp multiplied by the area of the equatorial plane (πr^2). That pressure force is balanced by the surface tension force which is σ times the distance around the circumference of the drop ($2\pi r$). Bachelor (1967) represented this balance as:

$$\Delta p \pi r^2 = \sigma 2 \pi r \qquad \text{(Formula 5.1)}$$

which can be simplified to:

$$\Delta p = 2\sigma / r \qquad \text{(Formula 5.2)}$$

where $\sigma = surface\ tension,\ and\ 4\pi r^2$ is the surface area of a sphere of radius r.

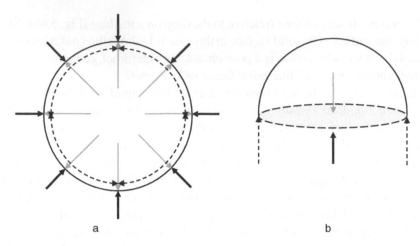

a   b

Figure 5.7 Forces in a droplet or soap bubble. (a) Atmospheric pressure acting from outside (black arrows), a slightly higher internal pressure acting from inside (grey arrows) and surface tension (dashed arrows). (b) The bubble or droplet cut in half along the shaded plane, an imaginary concept for the derivation of Formulae 5.1 and 5.2.

This gives us the formula for excess pressure inside the drop as a function of surface tension and radius, and tells us that the smaller the drop the bigger the difference in pressure, because the surface is more curved. Large drops have a smaller difference in pressure. Bubbles formed from liquids with smaller values of σ (e.g. detergent solution, compared to pure water) have smaller pressure differences.

Although blood consists of about 90% water by weight, the surface tension of blood is significantly lower than that of water (at 20 °C the surface tension of water is 0.072 N/m and blood is 0.06 N/m). It is not yet clear to the authors what component of blood reduces the surface tension relative to water, but it is likely to be glycerides and other components related to fat. Surface tension decreases as the temperature rises. Some typical surface tension values are given in Table 5.1.

If surface tension is the only force acting, a droplet will be pulled into a sphere. If some other force acts on it, such as gravity or aerodynamic drag, the drop will not be a perfect sphere. Aerodynamic drag can force a fast-moving drop to deform into a non-spherical shape. This will be discussed later.

Table 5.1 Surface tension of some common liquids. (Blood data from Raymond et al., 1996.)

Fluid at 20 °C	Surface tension at air interface (N/m)
Water	0.072
Mercury	0.49
Ethanol	0.022
Blood	0.051–0.061

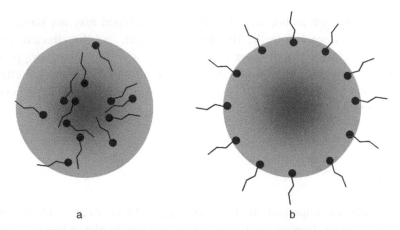

a b

Figure 5.8 Two droplets containing dissolved surfactant molecules, indicated with a black dot representing the hydrophilic head and a zigzag line representing the hydrophobic tail. (a) A freshly formed droplet with the surfactant randomly distributed; (b) a mature droplet, after the surfactant molecules have had time to diffuse to the surface and orient themselves.

As shown in Table 5.1, surface tension depends on the nature of any dissolved surfactants. These surfactants are usually organic compounds containing both hydrophobic (water-resisting) ends and hydrophilic (water-loving) ends to their molecules. Surfactant molecules will diffuse in water and adsorb at the interface between the liquid and the air (Fig. 5.8). This is because the surfactant finds its lowest energy position at the surface, with its hydrophilic head in the water and its hydrophobic tail outside in the air. Hence, surfactants will tend to gather at the surface of the liquid, although they take some finite time to diffuse to the surface and reach their full concentration.

Consider a surfactant solution, such as soap and water, driven through a nozzle as in a garden hose. As the water passes through the nozzle it forms drops and thereby new surfaces. The surfactant will take some finite time to diffuse to the surface. Where it passes through the nozzle and forms new surfaces, the surfactant concentration is low. The surface tension in this locale is very similar to that of pure water. For any fast process where the surfactant is not allowed to diffuse to the surface, the surface tension is very similar to the base solvent. In a slow process like passive dripping, there is time for the surfactant to diffuse and concentrate at the surface and, in that case, the surface tension of the mixture is strongly influenced by the surfactant.

In a pure liquid with no surfactant, the surface tension is always the same no matter how rapidly the surface creation proceeds; whether it is fast like a spray from a nozzle, or whether it is slow like a slowly forming drip, the surface tension is always the same.

It is hypothesised by the authors that the time-dependent surface tension described above may be relevant to bloodspatter. In processes that create blood droplets quickly, such as impacts, the surfactants in blood may not have time to diffuse to the surface before the droplets are created, and the effective surface tension may be close to that of water. In slow processes such as passive dripping, the surfactants may be present in high concentration at the surface and the effective surface tension is that measured in sessile drop measurements. This hypothesis has yet to be tested by experiment.

Viscosity

Viscous forces are important in the spreading of blood over a surface, in the formation of spatter droplets, in the spreading of those droplets when they strike a surface and in the forces in the air that give rise to aerodynamic drag.

Viscosity can be understood by considering the motion of individual molecules in a fluid. In Figure 5.9a, a fluid is flowing from left to right over a solid object. One molecule belonging to the fluid is shown, striking the solid surface due to the random thermal motion that all molecules experience. On striking the surface it bonds momentarily to the surface due to the short-range forces that keep liquids together. The molecule thus transfers to the solid object that component of its momentum which is parallel to the surface. The molecule will rebound and retain that component of its momentum that is perpendicular to the surface.

Through successive impacts of this type, the fluid in a layer close to the surface loses all momentum parallel to the surface and becomes stationary, relative to the object. This layer is one *mean free path* thick. The mean free path is the distance a fluid molecule moves, on average, before colliding with another fluid molecule. If the fluid is air at atmospheric pressure, the mean free path is about 10 nanometres (ten millionths of a millimetre).

The molecule rebounds and collides with a faster molecule further out from the surface (Fig. 5.9b). Upon collision there is an exchange of momentum, which slows the faster molecule and speeds up the rebounding slower molecule. This then slows a layer of fluid lying further than one mean free path from the surface. The net effect is to slow this layer of fluid, although it is not slowed completely to rest.

This process is repeated again one mean free path further out, to produce a layer a little faster still. In this way a series of layers is built up, getting faster each time until a maximum, called the *free stream velocity*, is reached. Above this all layers have the same velocity. The set of slow layers together are called the *boundary layer*. This is illustrated in Figure 5.10. Strictly speaking, the layers are not distinct and blur into each other.

The net result of the molecular collisions described above is that each layer of fluid has exerted a force on the faster layer above and the slower layer below. Each layer has attempted to slow down the faster layer and speed up the slower

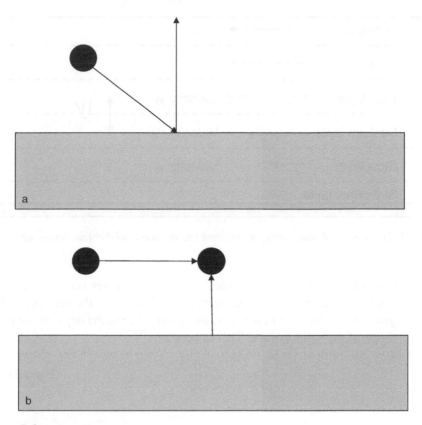

Figure 5.9 The origin of skin friction drag.

layer. This force is the viscous force. It is a shear force, in that it acts in a direction parallel to the surface and parallel to the direction of flow.

The viscous force is usually expressed as a *stress* force per unit area; units are N/m^2. The strength of the viscous shear stress, τ, depends on the viscosity of the fluid and on the velocity gradient in the boundary layer (Figs. 5.10, 5.11 and Formula 5.3). This velocity gradient is a function of the flow: the driving forces, the depth of the liquid and the shape of the solid surface. The viscosity of the fluid is an inherent property of the fluid and varies with composition and temperature. Fluids with long, chain-like molecules of large mass – like honey, tar or blood plasma, which contains long protein molecules – have high viscosity, as the long molecules collide frequently and transfer momentum from one to another efficiently. Similarly, fluids containing large particles, like red blood cells, have high viscosity.

The viscosity μ can also vary with the velocity gradient (shear rate), $\frac{dv}{dy}$, for certain types of fluids collectively called *non-Newtonian fluids* (Fig. 5.12). Such fluids follow the laws of Newtonian physics, but do not have a constant viscosity like the simpler fluids Newton described in his work on fluid mechanics.

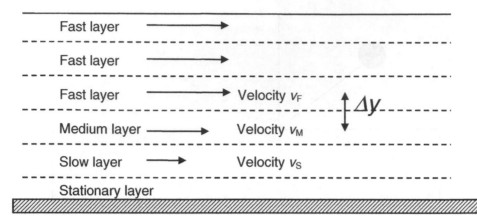

Figure 5.10 Layers of fluid moving at different speeds, over a solid object, setting up viscous stresses.

Velocity gradient, $\frac{dv}{dy}$, is the rate at which velocity, v, increases as one moves away from the surface of a solid object, increasing the distance to the surface, y. This velocity gradient is a function of the flow: the driving forces, the depth of the liquid and the shape of the solid surface. This is seen as:

$$\tau = \mu \frac{dv}{dy} \qquad \text{(Formula 5.3)}$$

where:

   τ = shear stress on a body = drag force per unit area
   μ = absolute viscosity (units: Pa·s or N/(m²·s))
   v = speed of air at height y from the body.

Viscosity is independent of shear rate for Newtonian fluids but not for non-Newtonian fluids (Fig. 5.12). Blood is an example of a *shear-thinning* non-Newtonian fluid, which means its viscosity decreases with increasing shear rate.

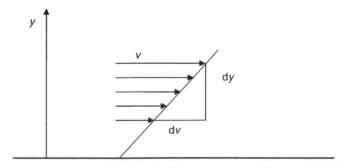

Figure 5.11 The velocity gradient in the boundary layer.

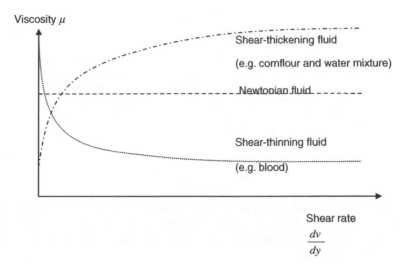

Figure 5.12 Viscosity as a function of shear rate for Newtonian fluids and two types of non-Newtonian fluids. Other types of non-Newtonian fluid, with different behaviour, also exist.

Drag

A body such as a droplet, moving through a fluid such as air, experiences forces due to the viscous shear stress and to pressure differences. These forces are usually separated into drag (the net effect of viscous and pressure forces acting parallel to the direction of motion) and lift (the net effect of viscous and shear forces acting perpendicular to the direction of motion).

Lift forces are very weak during the flight of spatter droplets, so this chapter will discuss only drag. The viscous drag force is called *skin friction drag*, and the pressure drag force is called *pressure drag* or *form drag*. A third type of drag, *induced drag*, occurs wherever lift forces are generated, but this will not be covered in this chapter.

Skin friction drag is simply caused by the viscous shear forces described above. When a droplet moves through the air, a boundary layer forms on the surface, with an exchange of momentum between the air and the droplet surface generating viscous forces as described above.

Pressure drag is caused by the pressure difference between the forward and rear faces of the droplet. The forward face experiences a high pressure due to the inertia of the air. This face is moving into the air and the air must be moved aside to allow the droplet to pass. The air has mass and therefore has inertia: a force must be exerted to accelerate the air. Since it arises from the inertia of the air, it is termed an inertial force and is given by:

$$F_{\text{inertial}} = A \tfrac{1}{2} \rho_{\text{air}} v^2$$

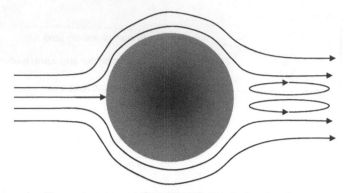

Figure 5.13 The paths followed by a fluid flowing around a sphere. On the downstream side (the right), the streamlines do not fully close behind the sphere, leaving an area where fluid is constantly re-circulated. This is called the separation zone, because the fluid here does not participate in the main flow.

where A is the frontal area of the droplet, the area it presents to the flow equal to $\frac{\pi d^2}{4}$ for a spherical droplet of diameter d, and ρ_{air} is the density of the air.

The equal and opposite reaction to this inertial force causes a high-pressure region on the forward face of the droplet. This pressure drag is enhanced by a low-pressure region at the rear of the droplet, 'sucking' the droplet back. This low-pressure region is caused by the air flowing past the sides of the droplet which, except at extremely low speeds, fails to follow the surface of the droplet right around the rear face (Fig. 5.13). This leaves a body of air trapped and is referred to as the *separation region.*

Both skin friction and pressure drag act to reduce the velocity difference between the droplet and the air. If the droplet is moving through still air, it will slow down. If the droplet is thrown into an air current, it will speed up to the same speed as the air.

The drag force is not exactly equal to the value calculated with this formula, however, because the size of the separation region varies and because of the viscous force. The drag force can be calculated by:

$$F_{\text{drag}} = C_{\text{d}} A \tfrac{1}{2} \rho_{\text{air}} v^2$$

where C_{d} is the drag coefficient, which varies with the speed and size of the droplet and the viscosity of the air.

5.3 Dimensionless numbers

In the world of fluid mechanics, dimensionless numbers have proved to be a useful way of describing processes over a range of different experimental conditions. Here we define two such numbers – the Reynolds and Weber numbers – which will be useful for our discussion of bloodstain formation.

Reynolds number

Pressure drag and viscous drag both contribute to the overall drag. Both increase in strength with increasing speed, but pressure drag makes an increasing contribution relative to viscous forces as speed increases, or as the size of the droplet increases. The relative importance of these two forces is estimated by calculating the Reynolds number Re as follows:

The inertial force or pressure drag is approximated as $A\frac{1}{2}\rho_{air}v^2$, and the viscous force approximated as $A\mu_{air}\frac{v}{D_{droplet}}$, where v is the speed, ρ_{air} is the density of the air, μ_{air} is the absolute viscosity of the air, $D_{droplet}$ is the diameter of the droplet and A the frontal area of the droplet. The velocity gradient $\frac{dv}{dy}$ is approximated as $\frac{v}{D_{droplet}}$. This inertial force is divided by the viscous force, the area A cancels and the factor of $^1/_2$ is ignored to give the Reynolds number, Re:

$$Re = \frac{\text{Inertial force}}{\text{Viscous force}} = \frac{\rho_{air}vD_{droplet}}{\mu_{air}} \qquad \text{(Formula 5.4)}$$

The Reynolds number is often used in fluid mechanics as it conveniently expresses changes that can be brought about by changing any one of the density, viscosity, size or speed of a system to achieve the same effect. For example, although the drag coefficient changes with all of these parameters, a droplet of 1 mm diameter travelling at 10 m/s will have exactly the same drag coefficient as a droplet of 2 mm diameter travelling at 5 m/s, if the air density and viscosity remain the same. Both these droplets will have the same Reynolds number. For this reason, drag coefficient C_d may be plotted against Re, as seen in Figure 5.14.

Weber number

The Reynolds number conveniently expresses the relative importance of inertial and drag forces. Where the Reynolds number is high, the inertial forces are strong and the viscous forces less important, and vice versa. Similar numbers can be calculated to compare other types of force. Surface tension keeps a droplet spherical, but if the inertial force is strong relative to surface tension, the front-and-back pressure difference will distort the shape of a drop. The surface tension force is approximated by $\sigma_{droplet}D_{droplet}$, where $\sigma_{droplet}$ is the surface tension of the droplet liquid. The

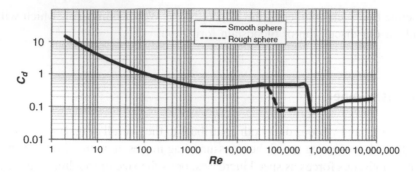

Figure 5.14 Relationship between drag coefficient of a sphere and Reynolds Number. The data for a smooth sphere is from Clift *et al.* (1978) to $Re = 3 \times 10^5$, and empirical data from Potter and Wiggert (2002) thereafter. The rough sphere curve is approximate empirical data also from Potter and Wiggert (2002).

inertial force is divided by this to give the Weber number, *We*:

$$We = \frac{\rho_{\text{air}} v^2 D_{\text{droplet}}}{\sigma_{\text{droplet}}} \tag{5.5}$$

A droplet will remain virtually spherical at Weber numbers less than 2. Above 2, the droplet distorts. At Weber numbers greater than 22 (or 13 if the droplet is suddenly exposed to the flow) (Wiersba, 1990), the inertial forces attempting to break up the droplet overcome the surface tension forces keeping it together and the droplet fragments into smaller packets of fluid. By virtue of their smaller volume, these may be drawn by surface tension into near spherical shapes which are stable with Weber numbers less than the limits mentioned before.

5.4 Fluid properties of blood

Blood is a complex, biologically active fluid with some important differences from simpler fluids like water.

The main component of blood is water (approximately 90% by mass in humans), and the density of blood (around $1050\,\text{kg/m}^3$) is very similar to that of water ($1000\,\text{kg/m}^3$), but it is the additives that give it its unusual properties. Whole blood can be separated by centrifugation into plasma and blood cells. Plasma is a Newtonian fluid (constant viscosity) and consists of water, dissolved proteins, fatty acids, glycerides and inorganic salts. The proteins, fatty acids and glycerides affect the viscosity and surface tension of plasma and, hence, of whole blood. When the clotting factors such as fibrinogen are removed from plasma, it is called serum (Krebs, 1950).

The white cells are present in small quantities and have little effect on the physical properties, but the red cells do. Red blood cell content is measured by centrifuging blood to separate the blood cells from the plasma and measuring the volume occupied by the red cells, which is called the packed cell volume (PCV) or haematocrit.

The red blood cells are principally responsible for the non-Newtonian properties of unclotted blood (Baskurt and Meiselman, 2003). In regions where there are low shear forces (usually due to slow local motion of the blood), the red blood cells form stacks or *rouleaux* (Fig. 5.15). These stacks cause the viscosity to increase. When the shear forces increase, the rouleaux break up and the viscosity reduces. Blood is thus categorised as a shear-thinning fluid. With the shear rate above a certain threshold, the viscosity becomes constant and, provided the shear rate remains above this, the blood behaves as a Newtonian fluid.

In the body, blood is maintained at around 37 °C. A constant exchange of water, nutrients, salts and cells with certain organs takes place. Once blood has left the body, the clotting or coagulation process begins. This takes some time – longer than most bloodstain forming events – so the properties of clotted blood will not be considered here.

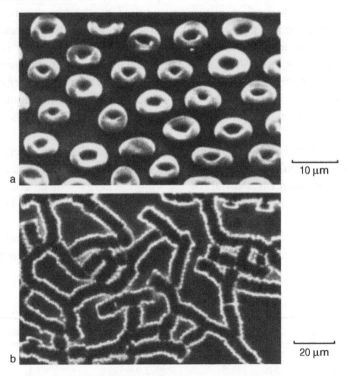

a

10 μm

b

20 μm

Figure 5.15 Electron micrograph of red blood cells: (a) isolated cells; (b) cells forming rouleaux in a region of low shear rate (Chien, S., Luse, SA, and Bryant, CA (1971). Hemolysis during filtration through micropores: A scanning electron microscopic and hemorheologic correlation. *Microvasc. Res.* **3**:183–203. Reprinted with permission from Elsevier.)

5.5 The creation of droplets

Energy required for atomisation

Bloodstain spatter patterns all involve the creation of droplets of blood from some larger volume. These smaller drops are projected onto nearby surfaces, creating the spatter pattern. The process of breaking up a liquid into droplets is known as *atomisation*. Atomisation requires that a new surface and, hence, a new surface energy, be created. The surface energy of a number of droplets (n), of a liquid with a given surface tension (σ), and all of the same diameter (d), is given by the formula:

$$\text{Surface energy} = n\sigma\pi d^2$$

This surface energy has to be provided by the process causing the atomisation. In the case of impact spatter, this energy is supplied by the kinetic energy of the impact. In the case of arterial spurt, the energy comes from the work done by the blood pressure that pushes the liquid through the arterial breach. In the case of gunshot wounding, the surface energy is supplied by the kinetic energy of the projectile, transferred by pressure and viscous forces as the projectile travels through the blood-bearing tissue. Generally speaking, if more energy is supplied, more, smaller droplets result. A large number of small droplets contain more surface area than the same initial volume broken into a small number of large droplets. Gunshot bloodspatter tends to form a very fine mist, comprising numerous very small droplets; whereas impact spatter caused by hand weapons tends to produce fewer, larger droplets.

Table 5.2 gives estimates of the mass, momentum and kinetic energy of hand weapons and some bullets, based on typical bullet masses and muzzle velocities for each type of projectile. Not all of the kinetic energy will be converted into surface energy, but this gives some idea of the energy available for breaking up blood into droplets.

The bullets have significantly more kinetic energy than the hand weapons, explaining the very fine spatter (small droplets), which is typical of gunshot bloodstain patterns.

Table 5.2 Energy available from various moving objects.

Object	Mass (g)	Velocity (m/s)	Momentum (kg·m/s)	Kinetic energy (J)
Fist and arm	5000	2	10	10
20 oz (567g) hammer	570	5	2.9	7.1
9 mm bullet (Luger P 08)	8	320	2.6	410
.22LR bullet (40 grain)	2.6	330	0.86	140
.303 bullet (150 grain)	9.7	844	8.2	3500

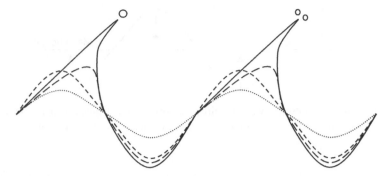

Figure 5.16 Growth of a wave on the surface of a liquid: a symmetrical, sinusoidal wave (dotted line) grows in amplitude (short-dashed line). It grows further and the peaks distort (long dashes) until the peaks break up into ligaments and droplets (solid line).

Fundamental processes of atomisation

Ultimately the mechanism which breaks up a body of liquid into droplets is usually a wave process. It begins with the generation of waves on the surface of a body of liquid. Under sustained application of the forces that initiated the waves, they grow in amplitude. When the wave amplitude is sufficient to pinch off small volumes of fluid, droplets are generated (Fig. 5.16).

Waves

All types of wave have a *restoring force*. Consider a wave on the surface of a body of liquid. Consider some disturbance, which raises the surface at some point (a peak). The peak will continue to grow under its initial momentum until some force slows it down. When it reaches zero speed, this force, should it continue to act, will pull the peak back towards the average height of the liquid surface. Having reached that average height, it will overshoot, due to its downward momentum and form a trough. If the force always acts to move the surface towards the average height, it will start to pull the surface in the trough back up, towards the average height again. Overshooting under momentum, the surface will form another peak. Such a process continues until it is damped out, with the kinetic and potential energy in the liquid converted into some other form of energy or dissipated. Such a process will produce a cyclic wave which persists for some time. To exist, such a process requires only a force which always acts towards the centre. This force is called the *restoring force* (Fig. 5.17).

The amplitude of the wave will change over time according to the relative strengths of the driving and damping forces. The driving force is that which causes the initial disturbance and which may cause further growth in amplitude if it persists. In ocean waves, the driving force is the viscous shear of the wind. Damping

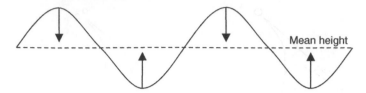

Figure 5.17   To sustain itself, a wave requires a restoring force, which acts in the directions of the arrows. The restoring force always acts towards the mean or average height.

forces are forces such as friction and viscosity which dissipate the kinetic and potential energy of the wave as heat.

Waves can be categorised by the type of restoring force. Consider waves on the surface of a liquid. Ocean waves typically have a wavelength (distance between successive peaks) of several metres. The restoring force for these waves is gravity; the weight of the peak causes it to subside and fill the neighbouring troughs. Such waves are called *gravity waves*. Waves of much shorter wavelengths (a few millimetres to a few centimetres), however, have surface tension as the restoring force. Such waves are called *capillary waves* and are the type of wave most relevant to bloodstain pattern formation.

If a jet or drop of liquid falls into a pool, a ripple is set up (Fig. 5.18). The ripples formed are capillary waves, and the excitation comes from the disruption of the surface from the falling liquid.

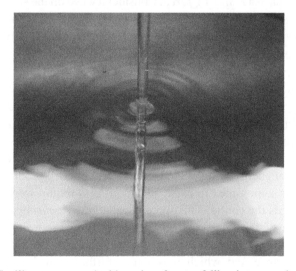

Figure 5.18   Capillary waves excited by a jet of water falling into a pool.

Viscous shear/jet breakup

Figure 5.19 shows a liquid film emerging at high speed into air. As the air moves over the liquid, a viscous shear force is set up. This force sets up waves on the liquid surface, which grow in amplitude until they start to break through the liquid film and form *ligaments*, which are line-like structures evident in the image. Waves also form on the ligaments themselves. These waves travel along the ligament and grow until the ligament breaks up. Finally, the resulting fragments are pulled by surface tension forces into roughly spherical droplets.

Figure 5.20 shows a picture of a jet of blood projected from a small round nozzle. Capillary waves are set up along the jet, leading to the breakup into small droplets. The driving force is the viscous shear caused by the jet moving against the air. Ligaments and droplets separate from the surface of the jet in an irregular process. Note the uppermost part of the jet is not broken up, because it is moving more slowly, as it was formed when the plunger was first being pressed. The process is irregular, because several waves of different wavelengths are present, each interfering with the others. The result is a wide variation in droplet size.

In this case the characteristic wavelength is less than a few centimetres, and the mass of liquid in these peaks is small and consequently gravitational effects are also small. However, because the radius of curvature of the surface is small, surface tension forces are strong. The waves are thus capillary waves controlled by surface tension.

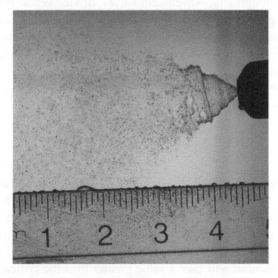

Figure 5.19 The breakup of a liquid into ligaments and droplets (courtesy E. Williams).

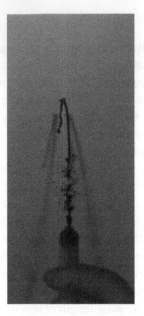

Figure 5.20 Breakup of a jet of blood from a syringe (Laber *et al.*, 2008).

Sheet breakup

Figure 5.19 shows a sheet of liquid produced by an industrial atomiser. Waves appear on the fan-shaped sheet of liquid. The waves close to the source are regular. Waves of different wavelengths move at different speeds, so short-wavelength waves may pass through long-wavelength waves, or vice versa. Waves of different wavelength also grow at different speeds. Thus the process becomes irregular further from the nozzle. Eventually as the waves grow in amplitude and the sheet thins, the waves begin to pinch through the sheet of liquid and break it up. Initially this forms isolated sheets of liquid. These break up further into ligaments and, as with jet breakup, these break up further into the droplets seen towards the left-hand side of the image (Fig. 5.19).

Bag breakup

Consider a drop moving through the air. The high-pressure region at the front of the drop where the air is impacting on it, and the low-pressure region at the back due to the separation zone, create a pressure difference which deforms the droplet into a bag shape. Surface tension opposes this, attempting to keep the drop spherical. If a droplet is moving sufficiently fast through the air or surface tension is sufficiently weak, the Weber number will take a value greater than the critical Weber number (13 for a droplet suddenly exposed to a flow and 22 for a droplet gradually

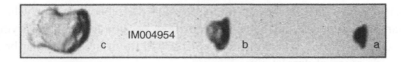

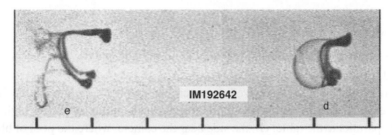

Figure 5.21 Bag breakup in water droplets (Luxford, G., W. Hammond, and P. Ivey, Modelling, imaging and measurement of distortion, drag and break-up of aircraft icing droplets, in 43rd AIAA Aerospace Sciences Meeting and Exhibit. 2005: Reno. Reprinted with permission of the American Institute of Aeronautics and Astronautics.)

accelerated), and *bag breakup* will occur. Figure 5.21 shows two examples of the progression in bag breakup. In both cases the drop is travelling from left to right.

Image (a) shows a strongly deformed droplet. Surface tension is weak compared to the inertial force which is distorting the droplet. The centre of the drop starts to blow out into a bag (b–c), which eventually ruptures (c). Waves grow on the rim and surface of the bag, due to viscous shear set up by the airflow over the bag, and the bag breaks up into smaller droplets. This process is responsible for breakup of large raindrops as they fall. Those that reach the ground have a Weber number less than the critical value.

A second example is shown in images (d–e). The formation of a bag is clearly seen in (d). In image (e) the bag has completely shattered.

Atomisation processes in some bloodspatter patterns

Arterial spurt

Jet breakup is relevant to *arterial spurt*. Arterial spurt gives rise to a jet of liquid moving against the air (see Fig. 5.20). This gives rise to waves travelling along the jet, and, because the driving force persists and the damping forces are small, the amplitude of the waves becomes larger as they move further away from the source of the jet. The jet breaks up into ligaments which will either break up themselves under the same forces, or be pulled into spherical droplets. The droplets will oscillate under surface tension, but, as drag reduces the speed of the droplet relative to the air, the driving force is reduced. When the droplet is near its equilibrium spherical shape, the surface tension forces are weak. The oscillation will die away due to viscous damping.

In an arterial spurt the wound through which the blood flows may have an irregular shape and there will be an unsteady flow, because the heart is varying the blood pressure through the cardiac cycle. This will result in an irregular breakup with a wide range of droplet sizes.

Impact spatter

Figure 5.22 shows the spattering of blood from the impact of a hammer on a pool of blood.

The pool of blood is squeezed between the hammer and the table. Being incompressible, it is driven out from underneath the hammer, acquiring high radial velocity, parallel to the table. On the side near the camera, where the pool of blood is shallow, instability in the advancing front of the blood causes it to break up into narrow, fast radial jets which leave thin radiating streaks on the table. On the other side of the hammer, the pool of blood is deeper and forms a thicker sheet of blood. The horizontal motion of this sheet is arrested by viscous and surface tension forces, and the sheet rises vertically upwards. Waves grow on the sheet, leading to variations in thickness that grow until the sheet is holed. The sheet then breaks up into smaller volumes of blood, which draw into roughly spherical shapes under the influence of surface tension. These travel in their original direction, modified by gravity and aerodynamic drag, until they hit the table or the back wall by the time the sheet has pinched through. Some ligaments and droplets are seen separating from the edge of the sheet due to the waves which are running along the rim of the sheet (b–c).

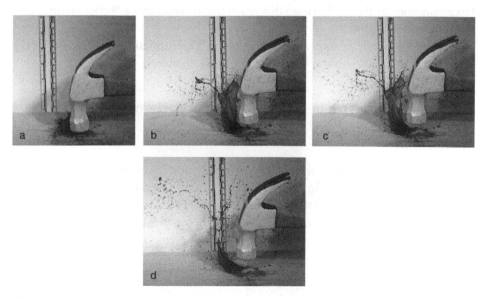

Figure 5.22   Impact spatter from a hammer striking a pool of blood (Laber *et al.*, 2008).

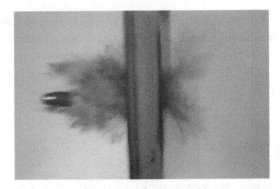

Figure 5.23 A.22 calibre bullet passing through a blood-soaked sponge (Laber *et al.*, 2008).

Gunshot spatter

Figure 5.23 shows an image from a high-speed camera of a.22 calibre bullet passing through a blood-soaked sponge. Fine spattered droplets are evident. These travel both in the direction of the bullet (*forward spatter*) and in the direction opposite to it (*back spatter*).

As it passes through the sponge, the bullet generates both viscous shear in the blood adjacent to the bullet path and pressure differences, between the blood in the pores of the sponge where it is compressed immediately ahead of the bullet, and further away where the pressure is atmospheric. There is also a low-pressure (vacuum) region immediately behind the bullet. The pressure and viscous force generate waves where the surrounding blood meets the bullet path. These waves grow until the wave crests break up into droplets.

Expirated blood

Figure 5.24 shows the phenomenon of bag breakup during the *expiration* of blood through the mouth. A bag forms (image a) and progressively breaks up, giving rise to very small droplets (b–c).

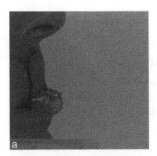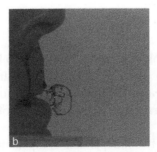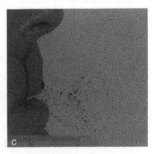

Figure 5.24 Bag breakup during the expiration of blood (Laber *et al.*, 2008).

Expirated blood droplets can also be produced by air blast atomisation, where air is forced by the lungs at high velocity past a film of liquid lining the inside of the nose or mouth (Denison *et al.*, 2011). At a critical point, waves will start on the surface of the film. These grow until they are stripped off by the airflow to produce very small droplets.

5.6   Droplet flight

Once blood droplets have been created by an atomisation process, they are usually projected through the air and land on nearby surfaces to form spatter patterns. Each droplet that flies through the air does so on a particular trajectory. This trajectory is determined by the forces acting on the droplet. In the case of blood droplets flying through still air, the only forces that need to be considered are gravity and aerodynamic drag (see Fig. 5.3).

The relevant formulae are:

$$F_g = mg$$
$$F_d = C_d A \tfrac{1}{2} \rho_{air} v^2$$

The *gravitational force* is the weight (mass times gravity), and it is a force that always acts downwards.

The *aerodynamic force*, F_d, always acts in the opposite direction to motion. This force is the product of:

1. the drag coefficient, C_d, which is a function of the shape and the speed of the droplet;

2. the frontal area of the droplet, A, the cross-sectional area as you're looking along the direction of motion;

3. the density of the air, ρ_{air};

4. the square of the droplet velocity, v^2.

So, to determine the droplet's trajectory we need to know what these forces are. Consider first the trajectory of a blood drop without drag. If there is no air, ρ_{air} is zero, so the drag disappears. We can solve Newton's second law $(F = ma)$, which describes the acceleration of a body in terms of its mass and the net force acting on it.

Force can be divided into two independent components: F_x, the net force acting in the x-direction (the horizontal direction) and F_y, that acting in the y-direction (the vertical direction). These forces are at $90°$ to each other and don't interfere with each other. With no drag there is no horizontal force ($F_x = 0$) and therefore no acceleration, so the velocity in this direction is a constant ($v_x = v_{x_0}$). (v_x is the horizontal component of velocity, and v_y the vertical component, where $v = \sqrt{v_x^2 + v_y^2}$.) Therefore, whatever horizontal velocity the droplet starts with, it will keep indefinitely until it comes into contact with something. The position of the droplet in the x-direction is the product of its horizontal velocity, v_{x_0}, and time, t:

$$x = v_{x_0}t$$

The vertical force is the weight force, which is the product of the droplet's mass, m, and the gravitational constant g ($F_y = -mg$). It is negative because it is a force acting downwards, which means it will accelerate in a downwards direction at a rate of $g = 9.81$ m/s^2. This means the droplet's velocity will increase to according to $v_y = v_{y_0} - gt$, and its y-coordinate – its height – will increase according to $y = v_{y_0}t - \frac{1}{2}gt^2$. This is the product of its initial velocity in the vertical direction, v_{y_0}, and time, t, minus $\frac{1}{2}gt^2$.

The droplet has a constant velocity in the x-direction and a gradually reducing velocity in the y-direction. A plot of these formulae gives the droplet's trajectory. Figure 5.25 shows an example of the trajectory of a 1 mm diameter droplet of blood (which will have a mass of approximately 5.5×10^{-7} kg, if we assume the density of blood is 1050 kg/m^3), launched at 4 m/s, at $45°$ to the horizontal. In the absence of drag forces this trajectory is always parabolic.

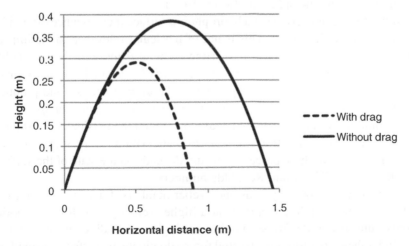

Figure 5.25 Trajectory of a 1 mm diameter blood droplet launched at 4 m/s at $45°$, with and without drag.

However, in real life there is drag. Under these circumstances the forces acting on the drop in the horizontal and vertical directions can be expressed by the following formulae:

$$F_x = -\frac{v_x}{v} C_d A \frac{1}{2} \rho_{air} v^2 \qquad \text{(Formula 5.6)}$$

$$F_y = -\frac{v_y}{v} C_d A \frac{1}{2} \rho_{air} v^2 - mg \qquad \text{(Formula 5.7)}$$

The horizontal force acting on the drop is purely the horizontal component of the drag force (Formula 5.6). The vertical forces are gravity and the vertical component of drag (Formula 5.7). An example of the trajectory of a droplet experiencing drag is illustrated by the dotted line in Figure 5.25. This trajectory is *not* parabolic.

5.7   Droplet impact: bloodstain formation

The last stage of the formation of a spatter pattern is the impact of airborne droplets on surfaces at the crime scene. In general, there are three processes that can happen on impact of a liquid drop. These depend on the Reynolds number of impact, the Weber number of impact, and the state of the surface. The Reynolds number of impact and Weber number of impact are calculated with Formulae 5.4 and 5.5, except that the density and viscosity used in the calculation are always those of the droplet fluid (blood) instead of air. The three possible processes at impact are termed bouncing, spreading and splashing (Rein, 1993).

If a droplet hits a hot surface or a hydrophobic surface it can bounce off and leave no liquid on the surface at all. This is not of particular relevance to the impact of blood droplets on typical surfaces of a crime scene. It is more likely that the blood droplet will spread and/or splash. Spreading gives a bloodstain that is larger than the droplet which produced it. Splashing is when the droplet spreads and produces a raised rim (crown), which breaks up into thin ligament structures or *spines* which fall down onto the surface and leave a wavy pattern on the outside of the stain. The spines may actually break off as separate droplets, which can be seen close to the parent stain. Which of these processes occurs depends on the state of the surface as well as the impact Weber and Reynolds numbers.

Bouncing requires low Reynolds and Weber numbers, for which inertial forces are relatively low. If a droplet strikes at a higher velocity, which means both the Reynolds number and the Weber number are higher, spreading and splashing can occur. Under these conditions the inertial forces dominate the surface tension forces, and the drop breaks up on impact.

Spreading

A droplet strikes a solid surface and spreads. However, the spreading is slowed by surface tension and viscous forces (Fig. 5.4). Hence, if the impact speed is high enough, this slowing has little effect.

Figure 5.26 shows a sequence of images from a 0.04 ml blood drop, falling 10 cm onto a cardboard surface and spreading. As the drop impacts the surface it deforms and spreads (b), producing a stain that becomes wider than the original drop. During spreading a wave expands outwards and the liquid forms a concave disk (c, d), after which the wave retracts a little (e). Surface tension forces are responsible for this retraction. Initially, the inertial force and internal pressure generated at impact overcomes that surface tension. Then, once these dissipate as the droplet expands, the surface tension causes it to retract. It does so in a symmetrical way, giving rise to a circular stain because this is a normal (90°) impact.

An empirical relationship between stain diameter and drop diameter has been suggested for blood droplets on a range of surfaces (Pasandideh-Fard *et al.*, 1996; Hulse-Smith *et al.*, 2005). Under conditions where inertial forces dominate and surface tension effects are negligible (which occur for many drip stain and spatter stain drop impacts), drop spread is a function of the Reynolds number only, which in turn depends mainly on the droplet speed and its diameter:

$$\frac{d_{max}}{d_{droplet}} = 1.11 \frac{Re^{\frac{1}{4}}}{2} \text{ for } We \gg \sqrt{Re}$$

In this case, surface tension is not so important in limiting the spread; although it is important in modulating the waves on the top of the droplet. What limits the stain diameter is viscosity. As the drop spreads over the surface, skin friction ensures that there is zero velocity in the liquid touching the surface and a higher velocity on the top of the spreading droplet. Hence, there is a gradient in velocity, and wherever there is a gradient in velocity there is a viscous shear force resisting that motion. Therefore, drops of the same size falling at the same speed, but with different viscosities, will spread by different amounts and result in stains of different diameters.

Splashing

Figure 5.27 shows a 0.04 ml blood drop falling 100 cm onto a paper surface. In this case, as the drop spreads, spines form on the expanding rim (b). These are due to *Rayleigh-Taylor instability*, which occurs as the result of the rapid deceleration of the blood–air interface along the rim of the spreading drop (Allen, 1975). This

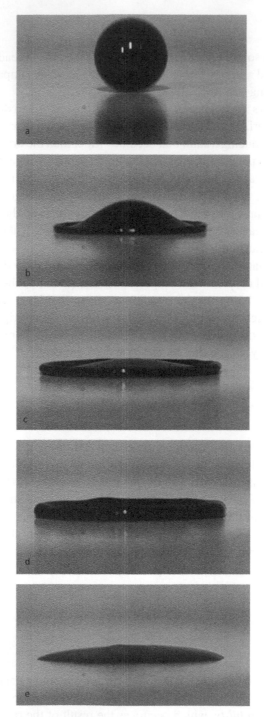

Figure 5.26   A 0.04 ml drop of blood falling 10 cm onto a cardboard surface (Laber *et al.*, 2008).

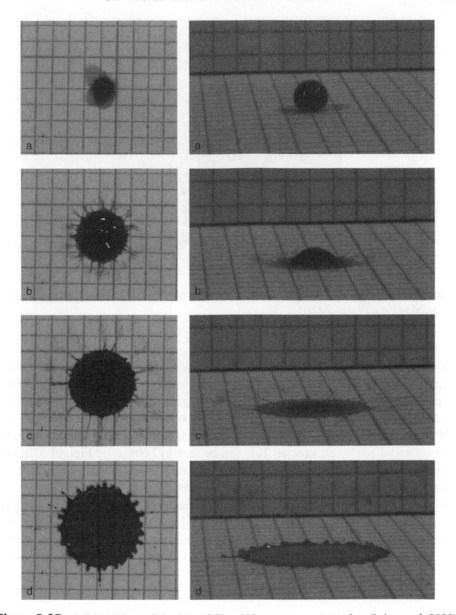

Figure 5.27 A 0.04 ml drop of blood drop falling 100 cm onto a paper surface (Laber *et al.*, 2008).

instability creates waves on the liquid surface that grow larger and form spines, which can, in turn, form droplets (c) – a process called *splashing*.

A criterion for whether a drop will splash on a given surface has been suggested (Stow and Hadfield, 1981):

$$ReWe^2 > k^2$$

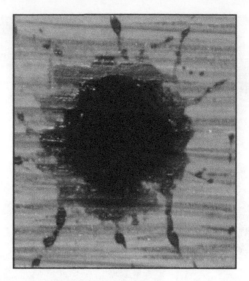

Figure 5.28 Bloodstain formed by dripping a single drop of blood from 100 cm onto a rough oak wood surface (Wells, 2006).

On relatively smooth surfaces, such as polished metal and glass, the surface roughness has an effect on whether a drop will splash (i.e. k is a function of surface roughness). For rough materials, including paper, card, wallpaper and textiles, whether the stain splashes or not depends only on the Reynolds number and the Weber number (i.e. k is a constant), which means factors such as droplet impact, velocity and diameter are crucial. This can be seen by comparing Figures 5.26 and 5.27, the latter showing splashing occurring on a rough surface when a droplet falls from a greater height and, therefore, with a higher impact velocity.

For very rough surfaces, such as concrete or a textured wood, which has a grainy surface in which the grain size is a significant fraction of the rim diameter, the protuberances on the surface produce irregularities in the rim. This leads to the irregular formation of spine lengths, spine widths and satellite droplet sizes (Fig. 5.28).

Droplet impact on wet surfaces

So far we have considered the impact of a blood drop onto a dry surface. But spreading on a wet surface produces qualitatively similar results. Figure 5.29 shows a sequence of images of a blood drop falling onto a wet film of blood caused by a single preceding drop. From the time of impact, a symmetrical circular sheet of liquid, sometimes referred to as a *crown*, forms, with spines starting to form around

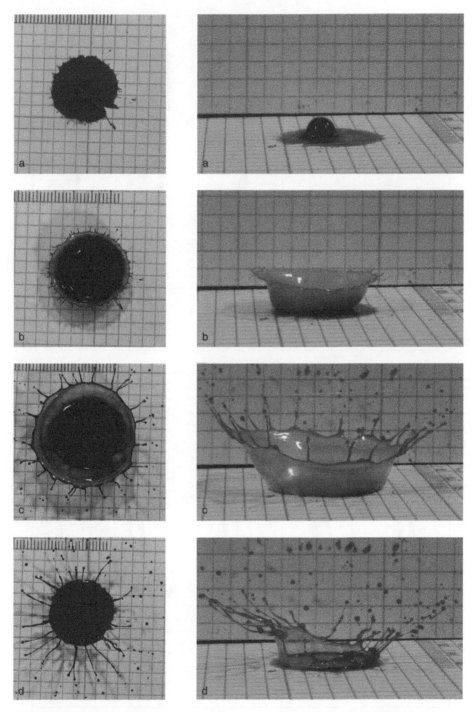

Figure 5.29 A drop of blood falling 100 cm onto an existing wet blood film (Laber *et al.*, 2008).

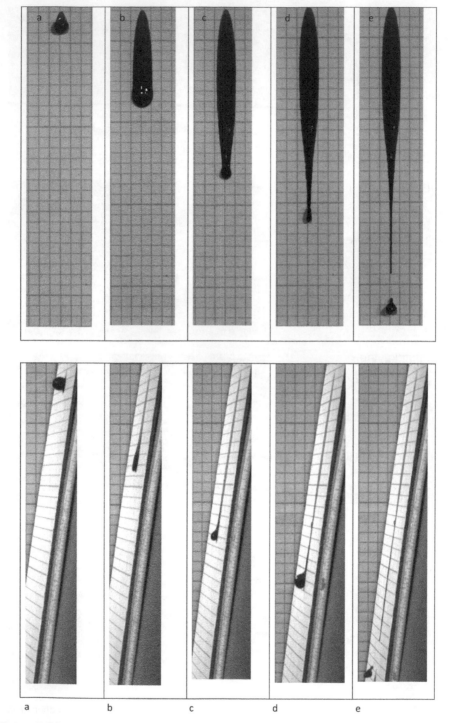

Figure 5.30 A drop of blood falling onto a paper surface inclined at 10° to the vertical (Laber *et al.*, 2008).

the rim (b). These spines become ligaments, which, in turn, form droplets which spatter onto nearby surfaces (c, d). This forms a characteristic pattern known as a *drip pattern* or a *blood into blood* pattern.

Droplet impact on angled surfaces

A blood drop impacting a surface at some angle other than 90° will produce a non-circular stain. Figure 5.30 shows a sequence of images of a blood drop impacting a paper surface inclined at 10° to the vertical. In the 90° impact, the momentum of the drop drove the spread of the liquid in a direction perpendicular to its original vertical direction. For an inclined surface, there is a significant component of the original momentum in the downward direction of the plane of the surface. This means the liquid spreads preferentially down the surface compared to the horizontal direction across the surface. This effect produces an elliptical-shaped stain (c).

In the final stages of stain formation, the last remaining bulk of the liquid is concentrated in the descending tip of the stain. Surface tension forces act to constrain this bulk in a near spherical shape to minimise its surface energy (c, d). For this steeply inclined surface, a small droplet forms and detaches from the stain, as a wave motion in the rapidly downward-moving, unstable lower section of the rim gives rise to the formation of a small droplet, which projects off the surface for a short distance before eventually falling and collapsing, creating a small secondary stain (e). The asymmetric shape of the stain is used by bloodstain pattern analysts to deduce the direction of flight of the original drop.

For other angles, there is a progressive change in shape from circular to elongated as the angle of droplet impact changes from 90° to some smaller angle, which is the basis for the well-known *sine law* used by analysts to deduce the angle of impact of an airborne drop from its resulting stain:

$$\text{Angle of impact} = \sin^{-1} \frac{W}{L}$$

where W = width and L = length of the bloodstain.

References

Allen RF. 1975. The role of surface tension in splashing. *Journal of Colloid and Interface Science* **51**:350–1.

Bachelor GK. 1967. *An Introduction to Fluid Mechanics*. Cambridge University Press, Cambridge.

Baskurt OK, Meiselman HJ. 2003. Blood rheology and hemodynamics. *Seminars in Thrombosis and Hemostasis* **29**:435–52.

Bevel T, Gardner RM. 2008. *Bloodstain Pattern Analysis: With an Introduction to Crime Scene Reconstruction*, 3rd Edition. CRC Press, Boca Raton, FL.

Chien S, Luse SA, Bryant CA. 1971. Hemolysis during filtration through micropores: a scanning electron microscopic and hemorheologic correlation. *Microvascular Research* **3**:183–203.

Clift R, Grace JR, Weber ME. 1978. *Bubbles, Drops and Particles*. Academic Press, New York.

Denison D, Porter A, Mills M, Schroter RC. 2011. Forensic implications of respiratory derived blood spatter distributions. *Forensic Science International* **204**:144–55.

Hulse-Smith L, Mehdizadeh NZ, Chandra S. 2005. Deducing drop size and impact velocity from circular bloodstains. *Journal of Forensic Science* **50**:1–10.

James SH, Kish PE, Sutton TP. 2005. *Principles of Bloodstain Pattern Analysis: Theory and Practice*, 1st Edition. CRC Press, Boca Raton, FL.

Krebs HA. 1950. Chemical composition of blood plasma and serum. *Annual Review of Biochemistry* **19**:409–30.

Laber TL, Epstein BP, Taylor MC. 2008. High speed digital video analysis of bloodstain pattern formation from common bloodletting mechanisms. *International Association of Bloodstain Pattern Analysts News (June)*:4–12.

Luxford G, Hammond W, Ivey P. 2005. Modelling, imaging and measurement of distortion, drag and break-up of aircraft icing droplets. Presentation at 43rd AIAA Aerospace Sciences Meeting and Exhibit, 10–13 Janary 2005, Reno, NV.

Pasandideh-Fard M, Qiao YM, Chandra S, Mostaghimi J. 1996. Capillary effects during droplet impact on a solid surface. *Physics of Fluids* **8**:650–9.

Potter MC, Wiggert DC. 2002. *Mechanics of Fluids*, 3rd Edition. Brooks/Cole, Pacific Grove, CA.

Raymond MA, Smith ER, Liesegang J. 1996. The physical properties of blood–forensic considerations. *Science and Justice* **36**:153–60.

Rein M. 1993. Phenomena of liquid drop impact on solid and liquid surfaces. *Fluid Dynamics Research* **12**:61–93.

Stow CD, Hadfield MG. 1981. An experimental investigation of fluid flow resulting from the impact of a water drop with an unyielding dry surface. *Proceedings of the Royal Society of London* **373**:419–41.

Wells JK. 2006. Investigation of factors affecting the region of origin estimate in bloodstain pattern analysis. MSc Thesis, Department of Physics, University of Canterbury, Christchurch, New Zealand.

Wiersba A. 1990. Deformation and breakup of liquid droplets in a gas stream at nearly critical Weber numbers. *Experiments in Fluids* **9**:59–64.

6

Fibres and textiles

Debra Carr

6.1 Introduction

Forensic textile science is a relatively young discipline; fibre identification is the most established component. Textile products of interest to the forensic scientist include individual fibres, yarns, fabrics, apparel and furnishings. Such products are often potential evidence in criminal investigations that have involved biomechanical incidents. Of particular interest is damage caused to apparel during an alleged incident. The nature of fabrics, such as fibre, yarn and fabric structure, elasticity, and fibre and yarn movement, can influence damage. Therefore potential evidence in textile products can be affected by poor handling (Adolf and Hearle, 1998; Taupin and Cwiklik, 2011). Evidence in textile products should be examined from the macro-level through to the micro-level (e.g. Pelton, 1995; Taupin *et al.*, 1999; Boland *et al.*, 2006; Taupin and Cwiklik, 2011).

Of key importance in such investigations is the correct and full description of a textile product using the appropriate discipline's terminology. Therefore, this chapter firstly provides a brief introduction to textile science terminology (for further information the reader is directed to standard texts e.g. Taylor, 1990; Tortora and Collier, 2000; Denton and Daniels, 2002); it then summarises and discusses pertinent peer-reviewed literature that involves the interaction of textile products with applied forces.

Fibres

A fibre is defined as 'Textile raw material, generally characterised by flexibility, fineness and high ratio of length to thickness.' (Denton and Daniels, 2002). In textile science, fibres are classified as being *natural* or *man-made* (manufactured). Natural fibres are further sub-divided into animal (wool, silk), vegetable (cotton, flax) and mineral (asbestos). Manufactured fibres are sub-divided into synthetic-polymer (polyester, nylon, polypropylene), natural-polymer (viscose, acetate) and other (carbon, glass) (Denton and Daniels, 2002).

Fibres may also be described by their length as being staple (short, distinct length), or filament (continuous). Fibre trade names, rather than generic names, are often referred to: e.g. Spandex® or Lycra® instead of elastane; Cordura® instead of nylon 6,6; and

Forensic Biomechanics, First Edition. Jules Kieser, Michael Taylor and Debra Carr.
© 2013 John Wiley & Sons, Ltd. Published 2013 by John Wiley & Sons, Ltd.

Kevlar® instead of para-aramid. If a product is identified on a care label as containing a fibre by its trade name, then clearly that trade name should be used in any report; otherwise the generic name should be used. Fibre identification is the subject of many standard texts and articles (Luniak, 1953; The Textile Institute, 1975; Hearle *et al.*, 1998; Robertson and Grieve, 1999; Carr *et al.*, 2008; Houck, 2009).

The chemical and molecular structures of fibres affect their physical and mechanical properties, including their interaction with liquids. More crystalline fibres are less absorbent. For example, flax is more crystalline than cotton and therefore less absorbent (Carr *et al.*, 2008). Thus, the way in which liquids (including biological fluids) interact with different fibres will vary.

Yarns

A yarn is defined as 'A product of substantial length and relatively small cross section consisting of fibres and/or filaments with or without twist.' (Denton and Daniels, 2002). In textile science, yarns are classified as being simple, composite (blend) or complex (fancy). Simple yarns contain one fibre type (e.g. 100% cotton), composite yarns contain two or more fibre types (e.g. 65% polyester /35% cotton), and complex yarns are often decorative in nature with irregular structures found at regular intervals along the yarn (e.g. slub, spiral, chenille and loop (bouclé)). A spun yarn is produced by twisting staple fibres together and is hairy in appearance. Spun yarns are manufactured from natural staple fibres, or from filaments that have been cut to form shorter fibres. Continuous filament yarns may be monofilament or multifilament and are smooth in appearance, but can be textured to induce a waviness or crimp. Yarns can be described as: single, ply (folded yarns), or cabled (cord yarns). Two or more single yarns twisted together form a plied yarn; if three single yarns are combined, then the yarn is a three-ply yarn. The combination of two or more ply yarns forms a cabled yarn, cables are combined to form ropes and ropes are combined to form hawsers.

Yarns can be twisted in two directions during the manufacturing process; these directions are known as S and Z twist. The direction of twist for a ply yarn is different to a single yarn to ensure that the yarn is balanced; that is, it is unlikely to snarl or untwist. The level of twist (number of twists per unit length) affects the properties of the yarn. A more loosely twisted yarn will therefore have fibres less tightly bound than a tightly twisted yarn. The fibres can slip out of the loosely bound structure. A more tightly twisted yarn will usually be stronger, more compact, less absorbent and less compliant.

Linear density is ' . . . mass per unit length of linear textile material' (Denton and Daniels, 2002). The SI units of linear density are tex (g per 1000 m). The production of a two-ply yarn or greater produces a resultant yarn that is thicker than might be first assumed due to a reduction in length caused by the twisting process. The two-ply yarn might be described as R36 tex/2: 'R' indicates a resultant linear density and

'/2' that two single yarns were combined to form a two-ply yarn with a resultant linear density of 36 tex.

Further information on yarns and ropes can be found in standard texts such as Lord (2003) and McKenna *et al.* (2004).

Fabrics

A fabric is 'A manufactured assembly of fibres and/or yarns that has substantial surface area in relation to its thickness and sufficient inherent cohesion to give the assembly mechanical strength. Note: fabrics are most commonly woven or knitted, but the term includes assemblies produced by braiding, felting, lace making, net-making, non-woven processes and tufting.' (Denton and Daniels, 2002). From a forensic perspective, fabrics of interest include wovens (shirts/blouses, suits, trousers/jeans), knits (underwear, jumpers) and home furnishings (curtains, carpets).

Fabrics are usually classified as woven (interlaced yarns), knitted (interlocking loops; stitches) or non-woven. Fabrics have a technical face and technical rear; the face has an improved appearance and is generally the outer surface of the product. Mass per unit area and thickness of fabrics can be important tools in matching fabrics.

The warp direction runs the length of a woven fabric, and the weft direction runs across the fabric. The sett of a woven fabric describes the number of yarns per 10 mm; e.g. 48×60 yarns/10 mm. Increasing the number of yarns per cm increases the strength in that direction, mass, abrasion resistance, stability and cost of a fabric. The edge of the fabric that runs parallel to the warp direction yarns is the selvedge; it is generally 2.5–5 mm in width, but can be up to 20 mm. A plain-woven fabric is the simplest weave that can be produced. Yarns are interlaced over and under each other at right angles. Plain-woven fabrics are reversible (unless a pattern is printed on one side). Examples of plain-woven fabrics include chiffon, gingham, chambray, cheesecloth, muslin, flannel, canvas and tweed. Variations of the plain weave include ribbed plain weave and basket weave. The characteristic rib observed in ribbed plain weaves is caused by the use of coarser yarns in either the weft or warp direction compared to the other direction. The rib is easily detected by running a finger up and down or across the fabric. Ribbed fabrics are often known as unbalanced fabrics. Basket weaves are formed by interlacing groups of yarns, the most common is the 2×2 basket weave (i.e. two warp yarns interlace two weft yarns on a repeating pattern). Twill weaves are characterised by diagonal lines on the surface of the fabric; for example, gabardine, chino and denim. The twill can be Z direction, or S direction. The simplest twill is a 2×1: each warp yarn passes over two weft yarns and then under one weft yarn. If there are more warp yarns on the technical face, the fabric is a warp-face twill. If there are more on the weft face, it is a weft-face twill. A 2×2 twill is an example of a balanced twill. Most twill fabrics are either warp-face or balanced. In a true satin fabric, one set of yarns forms the majority of the technical face of the fabric and the other the technical rear. A satin fabric in which the warp yarns form the technical face is a warp-faced satin, and one in which the weft yarns form the face is a weft-face satin. A variant is sateen, which is a durable cotton weft-face satin weave, often used for higher-quality bed linen.

Knitted fabrics are constructed by interlocking a series of loops (stitches); each new loop is drawn through those previously formed. Loops running vertically are wales; those running horizontally are courses. There are two main types of knitted fabric: (i) weft knits, and (ii) warp knits. In weft knitting the yarns run across the width of the fabric; each course is manufactured from the same yarn. Common weft knits are plain, rib and purl. Plain knits are easily recognised: the technical face is smooth with a clear vertical grain, whilst the technical rear is characterised by a horizontal grain. Plain knit fabrics tend to curl and are used to make underwear, hosiery, T-shirts, gloves and sweaters. Rib knits are characterised by ribs that run vertically; the rib is formed by wales alternating on the technical face and technical rear of the fabric. The simplest rib is the 1×1 (English rib); if two wales of stitches appear on the face and one on the rear, the fabric is a 2×2 (Swiss rib). Typical uses include socks, waistbands and cuffs. Purl knits consist of alternate courses of plain knit stitches and purl knit stitches. Therefore, each wale contains both types of stitches. A purl stitch is the reverse of a plain stitch. The simplest purl fabric is the 1×1, which consists of one course of plain stitches followed by one course of purl stitches. Alternative purl knits include 2×2 and 3×1. Purl fabrics do not curl. In warp knits, the yarns run vertically and each yarn forms a vertical loop in one course and then moves diagonally to another wale to make a loop in the next course. The yarns therefore zigzag from side to side along the fabric. The technical face is characterised by clear vertical stitches that are slightly angled side to side. The technical rear consists of slightly angled horizontal features known as laps.

Non-woven fabrics are ' . . . based on a sheet, web or batt of fibres bonded by mechanical, chemical or physical means' (Denton and Daniels, 2002). Typical examples include agricultural fabrics, dishcloths, disposable laboratory coats, surgical gowns and road reinforcements. The fibre types used in the manufacture of non-wovens are usually polyethylene, polypropylene, polyester and viscose, although medical end-use items can be manufactured using cotton. The fibre may be orientated: (i) in the longitudinal direction; (ii) in the transverse direction; (iii) in the longitudinal and transverse directions; or (iv) randomly. Non-wovens are classified into two major groups: (i) disposable (60% of the total consumption) – these fabrics are manufactured for single or limited use (e.g. surgical gowns); or (ii) durable (e.g. interlinings and agricultural fabrics), intended for prolonged use.

A number of other fabric structures that are not discussed in this chapter include carpet, felt, lace, coated fabrics/laminates, tufted fabrics and leather.

Dyeing and finishing treatments

It is important to note that dyeing and finishing treatments are routinely applied to fabrics and/or apparel, and that these can affect fabric properties including the interaction with liquids such as blood.

Colour can be added to manufactured fibres before extrusion (spun-dyed, solution-dyed or dope-dyed fibres). Colour can also be added to natural and manufactured fibres in a process known as fibre dyeing, or stock dyeing. Fibres are immersed in a dye-bath and then dried. Stock-dyed fabrics can be identified by removing an example of fibres from the yarn; the colour will be consistent along the complete length of the fibre. Yarns may be dyed as skeins (usually loosely wound), packages (yarns wound onto perforated tubes or springs), or beams (yarns wound onto large cylinders). Fabrics can be piece dyed. The fabric is passed through a dye-bath and absorbs the dyestuff. For a full discussion of dyeing, the reader is directed to publications by The Society of Dyers and Colourists (www.sdc.org.uk). Colour can also be added by one of various printing methods (Tortora and Collier, 2000).

A finishing treatment is '1. A substance or mixture of substances added to a substrate at any stage in the process to impart desired properties. 2. A process, physical or chemical applied to a substrate to produce a desired effect. 3. Properties, e.g., smoothness, drape, lustre, gloss or crease resistance produced by 1 and/or 2 above. 4. To apply or produce a finish.' (Denton and Daniels, 2002). Finishing treatments are classified as permanent, durable or temporary and include changes to appearance and changes to performance; a good summary is provided by Tortora and Collier (2000).

6.2 Fabric layers

Apparel is rarely worn as single layers; e.g. shirt under suit jacket, underwear under trousers and T-shirt under hoody. Consideration of the interaction of layers of apparel is poorly represented in the forensic literature; exceptions include Taupin (1999) and Daroux *et al.* (2010). In the wider literature involving impacts onto layers of fabric, the majority of articles discuss ballistic impacts onto body armour (typically comprising 20–40 layers of woven fabrics), which is outside the scope of this chapter. The response of different layers is affected by the amount of energy absorbed by each layer; higher velocity impacts usually result in holes in fabrics compared to lower velocity impacts (Joo and Kang, 2008; Laing *et al.*, 2008). Damage may be observed in lower layers caused by fibres from upper fabrics (Cheeseman and Bogetti, 2003; Laing *et al.*, 2008; Daroux *et al.*, 2010).

6.3   Fabric degradation

Fabric degradation begins with fibre processing (Slater, 1991). Once an item of apparel is manufactured from fabric, it is subject to increasing levels of degradation from environmental and use factors (Slater, 1986; Guoping and Slater, 1990). The major causes of fabric and apparel degradation include abrasion, extension, light (including ultraviolet light and daylight), weathering, temperature and relative humidity variations, ozone, atmospheric oxygen, wind, microbial and insect attack, dust, dry-cleaning, laundering, ironing, perspiration, water (fresh, sea, chlorinated) and chemicals (organic solvents, acids, alkalis and salts) (Dweltz and Sparrow, 1978; Warfield and Stone, 1979; Slater, 1986, 1991; Morton and Hearle, 1993; Gore *et al.*, 2006; Kemp *et al.*, 2009). The mechanical properties of fabric and apparel change with laundering. Similarly, washing will alter appearance and interactions with liquids (Sund and King, 1983; Slater, 1986; Gore *et al.*, 2006) (Figs. 6.1a,b). Thus, in any investigation, it is critical to: (i) identify fabric degradation and distinguish it from damage that might be forensic evidence; and (ii) understand how fabric degradation might affect any damage that could be of interest in a forensic investigation (Kemp *et al.*, 2009; Carr *et al.*, 2010; Daroux *et al.*, 2010; Carr and Wainwright, 2011).

6.4   Ballistic impacts

There were 41 shooting homicides in the United Kingdom in the year ending September 2010; this was less than 1% of all firearms incidents and approximately 7% of all homicides (Smith *et al.*, 2011). Seventy per cent of these incidents involved a handgun, and 17% a shotgun (Smith *et al.*, 2011). It is widely reported that close firing results in stellate damage to apparel fabrics; however, few studies exist in the forensic textile science literature discussing damage caused to apparel fabrics by bullets.

The effect of firing a Remington Nylon 11 .22-calibre rimfire bolt-action rifle, a Colt Woodsman .22-calibre rim-fire auto-loading pistol and a Winchester Model 94 .30–30 lever-action rifle at cotton fabrics (denim, broadcloth and jersey knit) and at distances varying between close contact and 6 m has been reported (Alakija *et al.*, 1998). Stellate damage did not occur with the .22 rifle; the .22 pistol resulted in stellate damage only when in contact with the fabric (close and loose), and the .30–30 rifle resulted in stellate damage only at less than an 8 cm range.

Poole and Pailthorpe (1998) compared impacts using a Winchester Superspeed .22 long rifle (solid point bullets at 350 m/s; hollow-point bullets at 400 m/s) on to apparel at contact and from a distance of 20 cm. The apparel tested was single jersey cotton T-shirt, single jersey polyester vest, plain weave polyester cotton shirt,

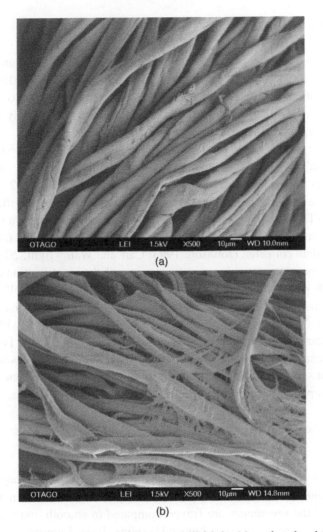

Figure 6.1 Effect of laundering on 100% cotton drill fabric: (a) not laundered (new); (b) after 60 laundering cycles. (Images: S. Kemp.)

warp-knit nylon slip and single jersey wool jumper. All shots penetrated the targets resulting in a ring of gunshot residue surrounding the bullet holes. The shape of bullet holes in the fabrics was more clearly defined for less-elastic fabrics; i.e. fabric structure affected morphology macro-features of the damage. Failed fibre ends were examined under scanning electron microscope (SEM); the appearance of individual cotton fibres was generally ragged, some wool fibres had longitudinal displacement of scales, polyester fibres had a variety of appearances – mixed but some 'mushroom cap'– and nylon fibres had 'mushroom cap' ends.

6.5   Sharp impacts

Sharp instruments are the most common type of weapon used in homicides in the United Kingdom (34% of all homicides in 2009/10) (Smith *et al.*, 2011). Approximately 80% of stabbings that occur in London are to the torso of a victim (Henderson *et al.*, 2005). Therefore, flesh and fabrics will typically be damaged by a sharp weapon during an attack.

Sharp impacts can involve weapons of convenience or of choice and include, but are not limited to, knives, screwdrivers, glass bottles, scissors, swords, axes, crossbow bolts and arrows, and razor blades (Ciallella *et al.*, 2002). Damage in fabrics (e.g. the dimensions) can reportedly assist with positive identification of the weapon used (Taupin, 1999). However, the substrate used to support a fabric during laboratory testing can affect the damage caused by the weapon in the fabric, and the variability of data collected (Johnson, 1993; Carr and Wainwright, 2011). Damage to individual fibres may provide some assistance with the identification of a weapon; however, such damage can vary among different fibre types (Adolf and Hearle, 1998). General guidelines for individual fibres are that: (i) scissor cuts result in pinched ends; (ii) knife cuts produce flat severances sometimes with a lip; and (iii) impact tears produce bulbous fibre ends (Hearle *et al.*, 1989; Pelton, 1995). However, researchers have reported difficulty in distinguishing between fibres cut with a knife or scissors, or among different sharp weapons (Stowell and Card, 1990; Pelton and Ukpabi, 1995; Kemp *et al.*, 2009).

Stabs

That blade morphology affects resulting severances in fabrics is recognised in the literature: blunt knives and knives with scalloped edges result in more fabric distortion, and the severances are frayed compared to smooth and sharper blades (Costello and Lawton, 1990; Monahan and Harding, 1990; Johnson and Stacy, 1991; Johnson, 1993; Adolf and Hearle, 1998; Pelton, 1998; Taupin *et al.*, 1999; Kemp *et al.*, 2009) (Figs. 6.2a,b,c and 6.3). However, severance dimensions in a 100% cotton jersey knit typical of that used to manufacture T-shirts were significantly affected by the type of support used in laboratory recreations of stabbing events (Carr and Wainwright, 2011). Severance dimensions in skin simulants are not necessarily the same as those in fabric coverings (Daeid *et al.*, 2008).

Slash cuts

Slash cuts involve a sharp object moving rapidly along a surface and can be divided into (i) chop and drag, and (ii) sweeping slash (Taupin *et al.*, 1999; Bleetman *et al.*,

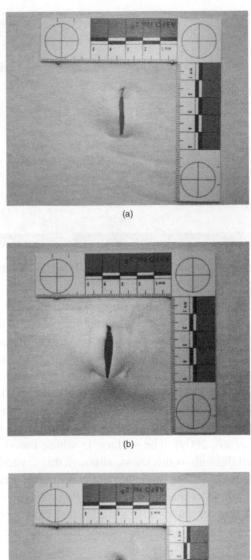

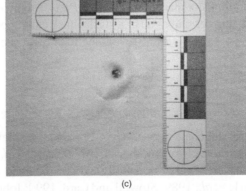

Figure 6.2 Difference in severance morphology in a 100% single jersey knit fabric due to different sharp weapons – note hilt marks: (a) kitchen knife with a serrated edge; (b) hunting knife; (c) screwdriver. (Images: S. Kemp.)

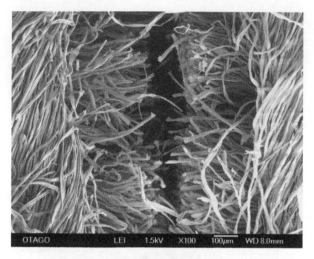

Figure 6.3 Planar array in stabbed 100% drill fabric. (Image: S. Kemp.)

2003; Fenne, 2005). Relatively little literature includes discussions of injuries and fatalities due to slash attacks; however, injured sites include the face/head/neck complex, the upper limbs, thighs and trunk (Ong, 1999; Bleetman *et al.*, 2003). Therefore, apparel may be damaged during a slash attack. Human performance trials using an instrumented blade ($n = 87$ assailants) indicated that the maximum force for a slash attack was 212 N (mean = 107 N), and the maximum velocity was $\sim$ 15 m/s (mean = 5.84 m/s) (Bleetman *et al.*, 2003). Similar velocities have been reported for stab attacks, but much higher forces occur during stabbing (Horsfall *et al.*, 1999; Kemp *et al.*, 2009). The surface in which the slash is made is not necessarily penetrated through its thickness, although this depends on the sharpness of the blade, the force used and the thickness of the surface; damage often starts and finishes with a clear point (Monahan and Harding, 1990; Taupin *et al.*, 1999; Causin *et al.*, 2005). Individual fibres damaged in a slash attack can reportedly be identified by a flat, clean severance, or by a flat severance with a lip (Pelton, 1995, 1998).

Cutting

Scissor cuts in fabric are characterised by stoppages or small steps which are produced by the opening and closing of the scissors (Taupin *et al.*, 1999). Fibres that have been cut with a pair of scissors usually exhibit flattened ends, often with a pinched section (Hearle *et al.*, 1989; Stowell and Card, 1990; Johnson, 1993; Pelton, 1995). However, two studies have suggested that there is difficulty in distinguishing scissor-cut fibres from knife-cut fibres, because use of both weapons can result in compressed and clean-cut fibre ends. In Pelton's study $\sim$6%, and in Pelton and

Ukpabi's study ∼15%, of scissor-cut fibres were correctly identified (Pelton and Ukpabi, 1995; Pelton, 1995).

6.6 Blunt impacts

Twenty-one per cent of homicides in the United Kingdom in 2009/10 were caused by hitting or kicking without a weapon; in comparison approximately 10% of homicides involved a blunt weapon such as a baseball bat, crowbar or hammer (Smith *et al.*, 2011). Human stomping reportedly results in a mean force of 6270 N; the force transmitted by a punch at 10 m/s varies from 2500 N to 3500 N (Mills *et al.*, 2003; Geoghegan, 2005).

Injury shape, for example bruises, can be examined to identify potential weapons used in assaults (Myers *et al.*, 1999; Thali *et al.*, 2003). However, blunt force trauma injuries can be difficult to interpret as they are affected by the impact force and the shape and size of the impacting object (Kimmerle and Baraybar, 2008; Whittle *et al.*, 2008). Fabric layers often cover the area of body being impacted. Therefore, apparel might provide valuable information about blunt force impact events in forensic investigations, even after the decomposition or healing of a victim's body; yet this topic does not seem to have been widely discussed in the literature (Daroux *et al.*, 2010; Figs. 6.4 and 6.5).

Quasi-static compression of fabrics has been discussed in the textile science literature; compression of a single layer of fabric occurs in three stages: (i) contact

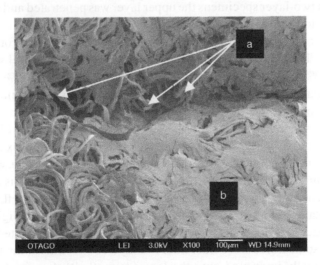

Figure 6.4 Single jersey knit impacted with a kerbstone impactor, 1.5 J, impact and scrape mode. Representative of tights/stockings/pantyhose (84% polyamide/15% elastane/1% cotton). Typical examples of damage: a = fibre severances, b = area of flattened and smeared fibres/yarns. (Image: E. Girvan.)

with protruding surface fibres; (ii) reduction in size of interstitial spaces between fibres; and (iii) through-thickness compression (Peirce, 1930; Matsudaira and Hong, 1994). Several fibre, yarn, fabric structure and finishing parameters reportedly influence the responses of fabrics to an applied pressure (Peirce 1930; Madeley and Postle 1999; Soe *et al.*, 2003; Behery, 2005). Therefore, the response of different fabrics may vary. The compression of multiple layers of fabric is influenced by yarn deformation, flattening and bending; and consolidation of voids (Robitaille and Gauvin, 1998, 1999; Chen *et al.*, 2001).

During an impact event, strain rate effects and the shape of the impactor are likely to be more important than during a quasi-static event. Reports on the effect of blunt impact events on single and multiple layers of fabrics are sparse; exceptions include Taylor and Pollet (2000), Laing *et al.* (2008) and Daroux *et al.* (2010).

The damage caused to apparel fabrics by impacts has been discussed for fabrics representative of tights, stockings and pantyhose, jeans, and sweatpants (Laing *et al.*, 2008); and for T-shirts and jeans or denim jackets (Daroux *et al.*, 2010). Laing and colleagues (2008) investigated apparel fabrics with reference to the use of lower-leg coverings in the prevention of pre-tibial injuries in the elderly. Even the low impact energies used (≤ 1.5 J) resulted in permanent damage to the apparel fabrics considered: e.g. impacts between 0.04 J and 0.59 J with a flat impactor resulted in yarn flattening; 1.5 J impacts with a kerbstone-shaped impactor operating in an 'impact and scrape' mode resulted in yarn severance, flattening and smearing (Fig. 6.4). Specimens consisting of single layers of fabrics were penetrated; in two-layer specimens the upper layer was penetrated and damage was visible in the lower layer.

In comparison, the work of Daroux and colleagues (2010) had a forensic textile science focus. Two fabrics representative of commonly worn apparel were investigated: (i) 100% cotton single jersey knit (T-shirts); and (ii) 100% cotton drill (similar structure to denim, jeans). Fabrics were impacted using two impactors: one representative of a hammer; the other a rectangular impactor which could represent a crow bar, as single and double layers (single jersey knit under drill; i.e. T-shirt under denim jacket). Fabrics were impacted, examined, laundered six times, dried, re-examined, and then impacted in a different position. This sequence was repeated until the specimen had been laundered a total of 30 times. All impacts resulted in a lustrous, flattened area visible to the naked eye due to fibre and yarn flattening; the shape of the damaged area reflected the impactor shape, but was slightly smaller than the impactor (Figs. 6.5a,b). Fibres and yarns in the impacted area were flattened and some fibres were fractured. For layered specimens, the upper fabric (drill) occasionally imprinted onto the lower layer (knit). Specimens laundered before impacting could be distinguished from specimens that had not been laundered before impacting due to more fibre damage in the laundered specimens. After laundering, damaged areas were no longer visible at low magnifications, but

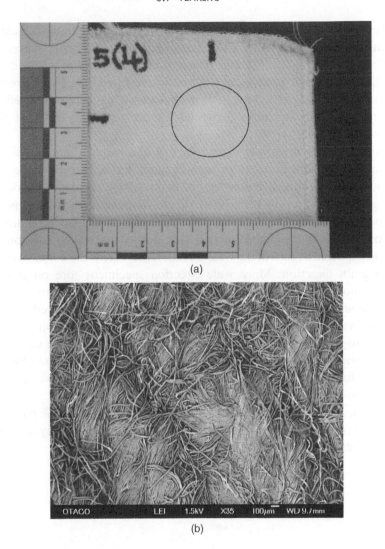

(a)

(b)

Figure 6.5 Blunt impact damage on 100% cotton drill, hammer impactor: (a) macroscopic damage (circled); (b) evidence of fibre and yarn flattening. (Images: F. Daroux.)

were still visible under higher magnifications. In some knit specimens, holes developed in the impacted area after laundering.

6.7 Tearing

Apparel may be torn accidentally during an altercation, or purposely when clothing is removed violently from an individual. From a forensic perspective, relatively little information has been reported in the peer-reviewed literature. Exceptions include tearing of apparel fabrics (Monahan and Harding, 1990), woven nylon fabric (Pelton, 1995), knicker fabrics (Dann *et al.*, 2012), and men's shirt fabrics (Mitchell, 2011), which have been reported in the literature. Tearing results in severances that are ragged and irregular in appearance, but can be affected by the fibre type and fabric structure. Some fabrics are reportedly difficult to tear (Monahan and Harding, 1990).

Dann *et al.* (2012) investigated the effect of fibre content and laundering on tear behaviour of fabrics used to manufacturer knickers (all single jersey; 100% cotton, 92% cotton/8% elastane, 92% modal/8% elastane). Fabrics were torn using a universal tensile tester to eliminate variation due to human performance. Specimens could be torn in both the wale or course directions, but specimens torn in the course direction (i.e. across the wales) tore on grain, whilst some specimens torn in the wale direction (i.e. across the courses) deviated from the grain direction. More wale-direction specimens tore on-grain with increased laundering. Force to initiate tearing varied among fabric types and between directions. Laundering did not affect the force required to initiate tearing, but wale direction specimens, laundered fabrics and cotton-rich fabrics were easier to tear. The torn edges of cotton specimens were more uniform than the other fabrics investigated (Fig. 6.6). Loops and loose yarns were observed in torn course-direction specimens; wale-direction specimens which tore on grain were more uniform in appearance.

Burying men's shirting fabrics (100% cotton; 65% polyester/35% cotton; both plain-woven) for as little as 15 days in either 100% sand or 100% clay resulted in a significant decrease in tear strength (Mitchell, 2011).

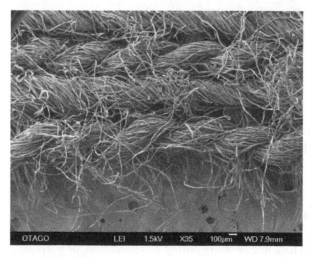

Figure 6.6 Torn single jersey fabric. (image: T. Dann)

Acknowledgements

The author acknowledges the following Masters candidates with whom she has worked, at The University of Otago (NZ): Shelley Kemp, Francis Daroux and Tanya Dann; and at Cranfield University (UK): Alex Wainwright and Jemma Mitchell. Scanning electron micrographs reproduced in this chapter were taken either by Elizabeth Girvan or under her instruction (Otago Centre for Electron Microscopy, University of Otago).

References

Adolf FP, Hearle J. 1998. Textile damage in forensic investigations. In: *Atlas of Fibre Fracture and Damage to Textiles*, 2nd Edition. Hearle JWS, Lomas B, Cooke WD. Woodhead Publishing Ltd., Cambridge: pp. 397–405.

Alakija P, Dowling GP, Gunn B. 1998. Stellate clothing defects with different firearms, projectiles, ranges, and fabrics. *Journal of Forensic Sciences* **43**:1148–52.

Behery HM. 2005. *Effect of Mechanical and Physical Properties on Fabric Hand*. Woodhead Publishing Ltd./The Textile Institute, Cambridge.

Bleetman A, Watson CH, Horsfall I, Champion SM. 2003. Wounding patterns and human performance in knife attacks: optimising the protection provided by knife resistant body armour. *Journal of Clinical Forensic Medicine* **10**:243–8.

Boland CA, McDermott SD, Ryan J. 2006. Clothing damage analysis in alleged sexual assaults—the need for a systematic approach. *Forensic Science International* **167**:110–15.

Carr D, Cruthers N, Smith C, Myers T. 2008. Identification of selected vegetable textile fibres. *Reviews in Conservation* **9**:75–87.

Carr DJ, Wainwright A. 2011. Variability of simulants used in the recreation of stabbings. *Forensic Science International* **210**:42–6.

Carr DJ, Kemp SE, Kieser J, Niven BE, Taylor M. 2010. Reproducing 'real' stabbing events in the laboratory: the importance of a textile science perspective. In: *Proceedings of Personal Armour Systems Symposium 2010 (PASS 2010)*, 13–17 September 2010, Québec City, Canada.

Causin V, Marega C, Schiavone S. 2005. Cuts and tears on a paper towel: a case report on an unusual examination of damage. *Forensic Science International* **148**:157–62.

Cheeseman BA, Bogetti TA. 2003. Ballistic impact into fabric and compliant composite laminates. *Composite Structures* **61**:161–73.

Chen B, Lang EJ, Chou TW. 2001. Experimental and theoretical studies of fabric compaction behavior in resin transfer molding. *Materials Science Engineering A* **137**:188–96.

Ciallella C, Caringi C, Aromatario M. 2002. Wounds inflicted by survival-knives. *Forensic Science International* **126**:82–7.

Costello PA, Lawton ME. 1990. Do stab cuts reflect the weapon that made them? *Journal of the Forensic Science Society* **30**:89–95.

Daeid NN, Cassidy M, McHugh S. 2008. An investigation into the correlation of knife damage in clothing and the lengths of skin wounds. *Forensic Science International* **179**:107–10.

Dann TJ, Carr DJ, Laing RM, Niven BE, Kieser J. (2012). Tearing of knicker fabrics. *Forensic Science International* **217**:93–100. doi: 10.1016/j.forsciint.2011.10.029

Daroux FY, Carr DJ, Kieser J, Niven BE, Taylor MC. 2010. Effect of laundering on blunt force impact damage in fabrics. *Forensic Science International* **197**:21–9.

Denton MJ, Daniels PN. 2002. *Textile Terms and Definitions*. The Textile Institute, Manchester.

Dweltz NE, Sparrow JT. 1978. SEM study of abrasion damage to cotton fibers. *Textile Research Journal* **48**:633–6.

Fenne P. 2005. Protection against knives and other weapons. In: *Textiles for Protection*. Scott RA (Editor). Woodhead Publishing Ltd., Cambridge: pp. 648–77.

Geoghegan T. 2005. A comparison of bloodstain patterns produced under simulated kicking, stomping, walking, and running. Unpublished MSc Thesis. The University of Auckland, Auckland.

Gore SE, Laing RM, Wilson CA, Carr DJ, Niven BE. 2006. Standardizing a pre-treatment cleaning procedure and effects of application on apparel fabrics. *Textile Research Journal* **76**:455–64.

Guoping B, Slater K. 1990. The progressive deterioration of textile materials. Part V: the effect of acid treatment on fabric tensile strength. *Journal of the Textile Institute* **81**:59–68.

Hearle J, Lomas B, Cooke W, Duerdon I. 1989. *Fibre Fracture and Wear of Materials*. The Textile Institute, Manchester.

Hearle J, Lomas B, Cooke WD. 1998. *Atlas of Fibre Fracture and Damage to Textiles*, 2nd Edition. Woodhead Publishing Ltd., Cambridge.

Henderson JM, Morgan SE, Patel F, Tiplady ME. 2005. Patterns of non-firearm homicide. *Journal of Clinical Forensic Medicine* **12**:128–32.

Horsfall I, Prosser PD, Watson CH, Champion SM. 1999. An assessment of human performance in stabbing. *Forensic Science International* **102**:79–89.

Houck MM. 2009. *Identification of Textile Fibers*. Woodhead Publishing Ltd., Cambridge.

Johnson N. 1993. Physical damage to textiles. In: *Police Technology: Asia Pacific Police Technology Conference. Proceedings of a Conference Held 12–14 November 1991*. Vernon J, Berwick D (Editors). Australian Institute of Criminology, Canberra: pp. 121–8.

Johnson N, Stacy A. 1991. Forensic textiles: the morphology of stabbed fabrics. *Australasian Textiles* **10**:32–3.

Joo K, Kang TJ. 2008. Numerical analysis of energy absorption mechanism in multi-ply fabric impacts. *Textile Research Journal* **78**:561–76.

Kemp SE, Carr DJ, Kieser J, Niven BE, Taylor M. 2009. Forensic evidence in apparel fabrics due to stab events. *Forensic Science International* **191**:86–96.

Kimmerle EH, Baraybar JP. 2008. *Skeletal Trauma: Identification of Injuries Resulting from Human Rights Abuse and Armed Conflict*. CRC Press, Boca Raton, FL.

Laing RM, Carr DJ, Wilson CA, Tan ST, Niven BE, Davis C, Bialostocki A. 2008. Pretibial injury – key factors and their use in developing laboratory test methods. *The International Journal of Lower Extremity Wounds* **7**:220–34.

Lord PR. 2003. *Handbook of Yarn Production: Technology, Science and Economics*. Woodhead Publishing Ltd./The Textile Institute, Manchester.

Luniak B. 1953. *The Identification of Textile Fibres: Qualitative and Quantitative Analysis of Fibre Blends*. Sir Isaac Pitman and Sons Ltd., London.

Madeley T, Postle R. 1999. Physical properties and processing of fine merino lamb's wool. Part III. Effects of wool fiber curvature on the handle of flannel woven from woolen spun yarn. *Textile Research Journal* **69**:576–82.

Matsudaira M, Hong Q. 1994. Features and characteristic values of fabric compressional curves. *International Journal of Clothing Science and Technology* **6**: 37–43.

McKenna HA, Hearle JWS, O'Hear N. 2004. *Handbook of Fibre Rope Technology*. Woodhead Publishing Ltd./The Textile Institute, Manchester.

Mills N, Fitzgerald C, Gilchrist A, Verdejo R. 2003. Polymer foams for personal protection: cushions, shoes and helmets. *Composites Science and Technology* **63**:2389–400.

Mitchell JM. 2011. Degradation of buried apparel fabrics. MSc Thesis, Forensic Modular Programme, Cranfield Defence and Security, Cranfield University, Shrivenham, Wiltshire, UK.

Monahan DJ, Harding HWJ. 1990. Damage to clothing—cuts and tears. *Journal of Forensic Science* **35**:901–12.

Morton WE, Hearle JWS. 1993. *Physical Properties of Textile Fibres*. The Textile Institute, Manchester.

Myers JC, Okoye MI, Kiple D, Kimmerle EH, Reinhard KJ. 1999. Three-dimensional (3-D) imaging in post-mortem examinations: elucidation and identification of cranial and facial fractures in victims of homicide utilizing 3-D computerized imaging reconstruction techniques. *International Journal of Legal Medicine* **113**:33–7.

Ong B. 1999. The pattern of homicidal slash/chop injuries: a 10 year retrospective study in University Hospital Kuala Lumpur. *Journal of Clinical Forensic Medicine* **6**:24–9.

Peirce FT. 1930. The "handle" of cloth as a measurable quantity. *The Journal of the Textile Institute* **21**:377–415.

Pelton W. 1998. Use of SEM in textile forensic work. In: *Atlas of Fibre Fracture and Damage to Textiles*, 2nd Edition. Hearle JWS, Lomas B, Cooke WD.Woodhead Publishing Ltd., Cambridge: pp. 406–415.

Pelton W, Ukpabi P. 1995. Using the scanning electron microscope to identify the cause of fibre damage, Part II: an explanatory study. *Canadian Society of Forensic Science Journal* **28**:189–200.

Pelton WR. 1995. Distinguishing the cause of textile fibre damage using the scanning electron microscope (SEM). *Journal of Forensic Science* **40**:874–82.

Poole F, Pailthorpe M. 1998. Comparison of bullet and knife damage. In: *Atlas of Fibre Fracture and Damage to Textiles*, 2nd Edition. Hearle JWS, Lomas B, Cooke WD. Woodhead Publishing Ltd., Cambridge: pp. 416–428.

Robertson J, Grieve MC. 1999. *Forensic Examination of Fibres*. Taylor and Francis, London.

Robitaille F, Gauvin R. 1998. Compaction of textile reinforcements for composites manufacturing. I: review of experimental results. *Polymer Composites* **19**:198–216.

Robitaille F, Gauvin R. 1999. Compaction of textile reinforcements for composites manufacturing. III: reorganization of the fiber network. *Polymer Composites* **20**: 48–61.

Slater K. 1986. The progressive deterioration of textile materials. Part 1: characteristics of degradation. *Journal of the Textile Institute* **77**:76–87.

Slater K. 1991. Textile degradation. *Textile Progress* **21**:1–158.

Smith K, Coleman K, Eder S, Hall P. 2011. *Homicides, Firearm Offences and Intimate Violence 2009/10: Supplementary Volume 2 to Crime in England and Wales 2009/10 2nd Edition*. Home Office, London.

Soe AK, Matsuo T, Takahashi M, Nakajima M. 2003. Compression of plain knitted fabrics predicted from yarn properties and fabric geometry. *Textile Research Journal* **73**:861–6.

Stowell LI, Card KA. 1990. Use of scanning electron microscopy (SEM) to identify cuts and tears in a nylon fabric. *Journal of Forensic Sciences* **35**:947–50.

Sund JL, King RR. 1983. Longitudinal wear study of four work shirts in ferrous metal operation; King County, Washington. *Fire Technology* **19**:163–9.

Taupin JM. 1999. Comparing the alleged weapon with damage to clothing—the value of multiple layers and fabrics. *Journal of Forensic Science* **44**:205–7.

Taupin JM, Cwiklik C. 2011. *Scientific Protocols for Forensic Examination of Clothing*. CRC Press, Boca Raton, FL.

Taupin JM, Adolf F, Robertson J. 1999. Examination of damage to textiles. In: *Forensic Examination of Fibres*, 2nd Edition. Robertson J, Grieve M (Editors). Taylor and Francis, London: pp. 65–88.

Taylor MA. 1990. *Technology of Textile Properties*. Forbes Publications, London.

Taylor PM, Pollet DM. 2000. A preliminary study of the low-load lateral impact compression of fabrics. *International Journal of Clothing Science and Technology* **12**:12–25.

Thali MJ, Braun M, Brueschweiler W, Dirnhofer R. 2003. 'Morphological imprint': determination of the injury-causing weapon from the wound morphology using forensic 3D/CAD-supported photogrammetry. *Forensic Science International* **132**:177–81.

The Textile Institute. 1975. *Identification of Textile Materials*. The Textile Institute, Manchester.

Tortora PG, Collier BJ. 2000. *Understanding Textiles.* Prentice Hall, Upper Saddle River, NJ.

Warfield C, Stone J. 1979. Incremental frictional abrasion. Part III: analysis of abrasion effects using photomicrographs of fabric cross sections. *Textile Research Journal* **49**:250–9.

Whittle K, Kieser JA, Ichim I, Swain MV, Waddell JN, Livingstone V, Taylor M. 2008. The biomechanical modelling of non-ballistic skin wounding: blunt force injury. *Forensic Science, Medicine, and Pathology* **4**:33–9.

Index

Forensic Biomechanics, First Edition. Jules Kieser, Michael Taylor and Debra Carr.
© 2013 John Wiley & Sons, Ltd. Published 2013 by John Wiley & Sons, Ltd.

Printed and bound by CPI Group (UK) Ltd, Croydon, CR0 4YY

09/10/2024

14571435-0003